Serving the Broccoli Gods

Serving the Broccoli Gods

True Tales and Tips from a Nutritionist on a Quest

Mary Purdy, MS, RDN

ISBN-13: 9781978078611
ISBN-10: 1978078617

Praise for Broccoli Gods

"*Mary's writing is honest, funny, and will inspire you to eat real food. I dare you to try not to fall in love with her quirky voice as she takes an honest look at her life as a nutritionist. You may just find yourself reaching for more quinoa and kale in the process, and liking it!*"
~Maggie Moon, MS, RDN, author of *The MIND Diet book*

"*Mary Purdy smartly bypasses the pedantic by sharing her own sweet, goofy, lovingly written story of forging a transformative relationship with food. You'll follow the tale for fun and punchlines, and be sent away with a brain full of comestible wisdom.*"
~ David Schmader, author of Weed: *The User's Guide*

"*Mary Purdy is pure genius when it comes to making nutrition information fun and accessible! Mary's personal journey will inspire you.... I'd like to make this mandatory reading for all of my patients!*"
~ Michelle Babb, MS, RD, author of *Anti-Inflammatory Eating Made Easy*

"*This one's a keeper.*"
~ Shauna Ahern, author of *Gluten-Free Girl*

TABLE OF CONTENTS

ACKNOWLEDGMENTS

Thanks to Corbin Lewars for her amazing editing skills; my writing group for very helpful feedback over the years; my parents for their never-ending support; and Keith Hitchcock, my champion and the love of my life, whose incredible talent and generosity keep me consistently inspired and ever blessed.

DISCLAIMER

The content of this book is intended for information and entertainment purposes only. It is not intended to replace or substitute professional heath advice or care, and should not be used for diagnosing or treating a health problem or disease. Please consult your physician before following any advice contained here. Never disregard professional medical advice or delay in seeking it because of something you have learned associated with this book. The opinions expressed in this book are those exclusively of Mary Purdy, and do not necessarily represent the views or policies of Arivale, Bastyr, Dietitians in Integrative and Functional Medicine, or other entities.

PREFACE

Is this book perfect? The best nonfiction read *ever*? Will it change your life and elevate me to the status of "life-changing author"? Probably not. (Although my mom would argue yes.) But my creative spirit is forever jonesin' for an outlet, and I have been writing over the years whenever I have had the time or inclination. This is the culmination of all that and I had a heck of a lot of fun writing it. I'm thrilled that I actually followed through with publishing it and even more delighted and honored that you are reading it right now. Thank you. I hope you have a laugh or two and perhaps learn a little something. Maybe you'll even discover a new vegetable/nut/fruit/bean and feel inspired to start consuming it on a regular basis. (Maybe as soon as you finish reading the first piece!) That would make me ridiculously pleased to the point of giddiness. Please write me and tell me if that happens, as it will make it all seem worth it. Photos of you and your new best food friend are welcome. It doesn't have to be broccoli.

THE MOMENT IT CHANGED

When I was four, my parents received a report card from my kindergarten teacher. The first line read, "Mary is a totally competent person." I'm not so sure about that. I have my good moments. And sometimes, I spend seventeen minutes searching for my house keys. The fourth line read, "Food is very important to Mary. If she doesn't have a good lunch, it seems to ruin her entire day." Now this I *am* sure about. When spicy chili and rice were on the menu (my absolute favorite dish as a young tot), there was an extra verve that carried me through my block-building and paper-cutting projects. When the offering was a tasteless bologna sandwich on generic white bread, I was prone to pouting and grumbling. Buildings went unbuilt. Scissors and pink construction paper lay dormant. (This still rings true—and if you don't believe me, you can ask my husband, who now witnesses my prolonged and palpable misery after a mediocre meal, whether it be at home or at a local restaurant.)

As I entered elementary and middle school, my enthusiasm for scrumptious meals continued, but it was joined by an interest in how food affected health. I would occasionally peruse the health section of my parents' *New York Times** (shout-out to *Times* writer Jane Brody) and read with great curiosity how eating broccoli might extend my existence.

At ten years old, I came across a book on CPR that my older brother had been required to read for a course. Reading the book convinced me that cardiac arrest was imminent or at least a possibility. My hope was

---

* It is possible that I am remembering myself perusing the *New York Times* when in actuality it may have been my mom cutting out articles and putting them on my dresser.

1

that by eating broccoli and whole-wheat pasta, I might help prevent an early demise. Don't get me wrong—like most ten-year-olds, I loathed and refused zucchini and spinach and once was bribed by my mom with five dollars to finish the peas on my plate. (I hadn't read anything about the death-defying power of peas; otherwise I might have been more inclined to gobble them up.) I was also known to consume large quantities of Swedish Fish and an entire pan of Rice Krispies treats in one sitting. I associated sugar with cavities, which might necessitate a large needle jabbing into your gums but as far as I knew didn't kill you.

My keen interest in staving off death for as long as possible fueled my zeal both for eating well and for learning about nutrition. While in high school, I was often scoffed at for eating apples instead of chips or salad instead of fries. (I sometimes ponder whether McDonald's healthy options were inspired by my teenage resolve.)

Although fascinated by nutrition, I was even more passionate about theater and acting. Therefore, I chose to major in acting while in college and made acting my career in New York City for eleven years. (Please stay tuned for my next book on the joys of "trying to make it.") Nonetheless, to satiate my nutritional desires during this time, I read countless magazine articles on partially hydrogenated oils, the benefits of juicing, and Coenzyme Q10. I kept an eye on the contents of my kitchen cabinets and made efforts to eat as many healthy foods as I could find and afford. I attended health fairs, bought a $400 blender, started taking every supplement I read about, and even wound up assisting in the marketing plan of a nutritionist when I was between gigs. She got me going hard on quinoa, kale, and cashew cream—all of which fell under the category of foods that had the potential to extend your life and made your skin look nice as a by-product. I was hooked.

This would be a good time to touch upon another obsession of mine: wrinkles. Have I mentioned that I was also somewhat infatuated with doing what I could to avoid wrinkles for as long as possible? This began at age fifteen when I heard about the power of Noxzema face wash, Sea Breeze toner, and apricot exfoliating scrub, which I slathered on morning and night until my face took on the gleam of a waxed cucumber and smelled like antiseptic jam. Of course, the need for a flawless epidermis was also strongly fueled by that Hollywood pressure to remain ageless and devoid of pores and pimples if you ever wanted to land a job that didn't involve playing a witch in *Macbeth* or the goofy and perpetually single next-door neighbor. When I understood that healthy food not only made my innards extra groovy but my outer layer über glowy, I had no issue with replacing cream soda with kale smoothies.

In 2003, my dad came down with a very serious disease called meningococcemia, which landed him in the hospital for months and nearly killed him. He lost the lower half of both of his legs as well as a large chunk of weight—to which his already skinny frame did not need to say goodbye. His appetite was almost nonexistent, and he was being partially fed via a tube in his stomach (some delicious slurry, I'm sure, of very high-quality soybean oil, corn syrup, and hydrolyzed whey proteins). While I knew that broccoli would not help my dad sprout new legs, I did believe that food might have something to do with the rate at which he healed and might positively or negatively affect his outcome.

I almost went into cardiac arrest when the hospital dietitian took me aside and said, "Your father has lost a lot of weight. If he wants a Big Mac, give him a Big Mac. He just needs to gain weight."

Two things went through my mind. Number one, my dad had never eaten a Big Mac in his entire life, nor would he even dream of setting foot in a McDonald's (even for apples or a side salad). Fast food was frowned upon in the Purdy household, although I periodically begged my mom for one of those talcum-powdery strawberry shakes when I was nine. "Absolutely not, Mary!" came the reply from my unbudging mother. The food was deemed "junk," the containers "cheap looking," and the atmosphere "depressing."

Number two, although I wasn't a doctor or even a dietitian, I was pretty sure that recommending a Big Mac for someone whose organs had shut down and whose body was desperately trying to repair necrotic skin was ill advised and possibly irresponsible. I was sure he could gain weight without resorting to eating a poor-quality beef slab with mayonnaise on a trans-fatty white-flour sesame seed bun.* I cannot remember exactly how I responded to this woman with a master's degree in clinical nutrition who worked at a highly regarded hospital in New York City, but it may have been something like, "Whuh?" accompanied by a thick crease in my forehead that likely began my aging process. I had to double up on the Noxzema that night.

That was the moment when things just clicked. Here was my clear sign from the Broccoli Gods that it was time to make a definitive change. I admit my career in the theater (although it sounds very glamorous, I know!) had proved to be somewhat heartbreaking, soul sucking, disappointing, weathering, and ego draining. I had heard enough "We're going a different direction" and "I'll contact you when we have something right for you" that the starry-eyed vigor of my twenty-two-year-old self had become a teary-eyed dimness at thirty-three. I was left with a sense of uselessness, like a VCR in the age of DVDs.

But as a dietitian, I could be useful. I felt determined that no other family with a skinny and appetite-challenged loved one in the hospital would ever be advised or encouraged to consume a Whopper before discussing healthier options first, like luscious and groovy fat-containing avocados and walnuts. Thank you, reckless dietitian! Your words changed my life.

Before I knew it, I had enrolled in a biology class at LaGuardia Community College. (My lab partner was half my age, but she really knew how to rip the fascia out of a cat corpse!) Next up: organic chemistry, anatomy, and physiology. I had never considered myself a math or science person. I chose the undergrad college I had gone to (Oberlin) based on the fact that there were no requirements to take classes in these departments. "Who is ever going to use geometry again?" I remember moaning. "Why on earth should I care about Bunsen burners? I'm an artist!" I traipsed around campus in my flower-print corduroy overalls

---

* As a dietitian myself now, I know how critical it is not to lose weight when haggling with a serious disease like cancer. Unintentional weight loss is one of the greatest predictors of poor outcomes.

and a "This is what a feminist looks like" T-shirt with my copy of Elie Wiesel's *Night* under one arm and a temporary tattoo of Buddha on the other. My whole college career was predicated on the fact that I could get academic credit for creating a comedy improv group and playing Mrs. Lovett in *Sweeney Todd* during our self-designed January winter term.

Now I was sitting in large lecture halls, brain buzzing with words like *cofactors, acetyl groups,* and *ventricles*—and loving it, despite the chirps in my head of "Are you really doing this?" This may sound odd, but I had the distinct sensation of what I can only describe as a cellular shift, as if my core identity was a muscle that I could actually see and feel pulsating, growing new blood vessels (mutating, perhaps?), and forming itself into something different from what I knew. It was similar to the feeling I had when I realized that I could read, or that I was one day going to grow boobs, or how I imagine Helen Keller might have felt when she finally got it that all that friggin' wet stuff getting pumped out of that contraption and all over her gingham dress by Annie Sullivan was "water." Food wasn't just something I happily gobbled down three times daily (or more, if I'm being realistic. Come on, snacks!), it was something I could study and apply to life. It wasn't just the thing that helped me live but could be the thing that helped me make my living.

While my dad learned how to use his fancy new prosthetic legs, I learned all about the bones, tendons, ligaments, and blood vessels involved in the real ones that he had lost. While he regained the strength and weight needed to get back to his life, I regained the confidence and drive to move forward with mine. The Broccoli Gods smiled, and I built them an informal altar in my kitchen next to the Roach Motel.

Get Your Happy Healthy Weight Gain Right Here!

If you or a family member is struggling and needs to find an easy way to gain weight, please allow me to suggest something besides Boost or Ensure. While being named after very comforting verbs, these shakes consist of subpar ingredients and taste a bit like liquefied chalk mixed with Hershey's syrup.

The labels boast 240 calories, which includes 10 grams of protein, 3 grams of fiber, and all kinds of added vitamins and minerals. Sounds simple, yes? Well, the fats and protein come respectively from low-quality corn oil (yummy!) and isolated soy and broken-down whey, and the carbs from sugar and corn-derived maltodextrin. Fats are not just calories; they have an impact on your body like helping to dictate how your body responds to inflammation. Not all protein is the same. Quality and form matter. Refined sugar can be fun (who hasn't enjoyed a packet of Skittles in life?) but is not the optimal way to put on pounds.

These products also have sneaky code words for their additives, which they refer to as "supporting ingredients." For example, "potassium hydroxide" (used in batteries, biodiesel, and soft soap, thus perfect for a healthy beverage!) is lovingly titled a "balancing agent." I get it; if energy and creativity are low, and you want to just go ahead and buy something that has an easy 240 calories, I can recommend a very similar product called Orgain (www.orgain.com), a healthier version of a high-calorie beverage. However, if you have enough oomph to open a jar of peanut butter, peel a banana, and assemble some additional ingredients into a blender, you can also make a very quick and easy smoothie and pop a high-quality multivitamin for extra insurance.

Easy High-Cal Smoothie by Mary Purdy

1 banana (~80 calories + 3 grams of fiber)

½ cup 2 percent vanilla yogurt (~100 calories + 5 grams of protein)

2 tablespoons of peanut/almond butter (180 calories with 8 grams of protein and 2 grams of fiber)

½ cup of water or choose your milk (an extra 50 calories depending on what you choose)

Put ingredients in blender and press blend/mix or whatever verb on your contraption gets blades turning vigorously enough to transform a banana into a beverage.

Total: ~350 calories (give or take), ~13 grams of protein, ~18grams of fat.

Simple and battery-acid-ingredient free! Plus, who doesn't love bananas and peanut butter? Throw a tablespoon of cocoa powder or a couple squares of dark chocolate in there and voila! Your peanut-butter cup smoothie is ready.

THE ROAD TO KALE

I t was settled. At thirty-three years old, I let go of eleven years of a life of pounding the theatrical pavement in New York City (or what felt like signing up for weekly heartbreak for my soul) and decided to pursue a life in nutrition where I wouldn't need a one-woman show (of which I had two) or an agent (of which I had none) to land a job.* It didn't seem like the most unlikely of career leaps, since my fascination with food had followed me around like a puppy for years, waiting for me to notice that she was now a full-grown Lassie eager to help save the day.

I learned about a graduate program in clinical nutrition at Bastyr University in Seattle, a university renowned for its innovative and integrative approach to medicine. I celebrated with a massive kale smoothie when I was accepted and packed up my New York City apartment in preparation for the seven-day drive to the rainiest and greenest city in the nation.

My boyfriend at the time, Todd, outfitted me with a *Healthy Highways* guidebook to help me navigate my way to nutritious pit stops along the journey: a vegan café in Columbus, Ohio; a raw foods juice bar in Lincoln, Nebraska; and a farmers market in Twin Falls, Idaho. I giggled, cooed, and sang my whole way there, checking my gut constantly for a feeling of doubt, which never appeared. I felt sure that Jane Brody would be proud, my kindergarten teacher would totally understand, and my dad's future meningococcemia-having cohorts would kick up their prosthetic heels in gratitude.

---

* Although, stay tuned about that one-woman nutritional show. You might be surprised. Food can be funny. Hee hee.

I knew that my now official *academic* devotion and commitment to broccoli and other members of the cruciferous vegetable family would extend not only my own life but also the lives of many others. Finally, I would be entering into a community where I would meet fellow colleagues who gleaned the same level of joy from a grain bowl that I did.

Arriving in Seattle in late June was like landing in Oz, with a landscape of brilliant color, random singing everywhere, cheery people on the street who said hello when you passed, and an amazing hairdresser who convinced me that my hair was meant to be curly—and made it so. For the following month, as I set up my house (with…gasp…a fireplace and kitchen that was not the size of a closet!), my spirits were so elevated that I decided to watch every horribly sad movie that I hadn't yet seen: *Hotel Rwanda, Maria Full of Grace, Dancer in the Dark.* There was no subject so depressing that it could stop the constant smile on my face or the pep in my step as I biked to yoga, wandered around my new food co-op, took late-night walks in what felt like daylight (bless you Pacific Northwest!) and devoured my intensive summer biochemistry class from the front row every day. That's right: this artsy hippie couldn't stop yammering on about the molecular basis for human life.

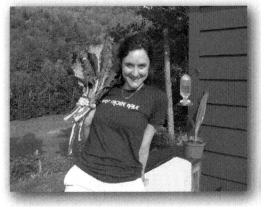

Before I left, Todd, told me that I had to meet his dear friend from graduate drama school, Keith, who also lived in Seattle. "You two will totally get along!" His endorsement meant a lot when I was going to be new to town, on my own, entrenched in school, and needing a guarantee that any potential friendship would be worth the pockets of time between "Nutritional Assessment" and "Disease Pathology."

I met Keith when he showed up on my doorstep with fresh-picked blueberries at the first late-summer party I threw to celebrate the twenty-seven new friends I had made through my graduate program and the neighborhood. That night, while we sat together on lawn chairs at an outdoor movie postparty, laughing at the same funny moments and munching on Bing cherries and Trader Joe's popcorn, I thought, "This guy's going to be one of my best friends here."

With the tacit understanding of a platonic relationship solidified by our respective relationships with and respect for Todd, we quickly became best buds. I didn't consider Keith my type anyway. Being on the tall and skinny side myself, I went for slim fellas who towered over me, enabling me to feel dainty and feminine. Keith's eyes met my eyebrows. I was partial to a little facial hair (except on my *own* chinny chin chin, of course). Keith was beardless. Our friendship deepened easily and without expectation. He was also a theater artist in transition, a meditator, a listener, and a dedicated vegetarian who subsisted on soy—which, it turned out after some informal nutritional counseling/detective work, was the culprit in some digestive distress he was experiencing. You might say he was my first "official" patient before I got my master's degree. (Don't tell the Commission on Dietetic Registration.) We saw dozens of alternative theatre shows together, took road trips to fringe festivals, and created a duo act: the foreign couple "Yostenko and Iscratcha from Yomenia." I tried to figure out ways to set him up with my nettle-tea-sipping and grass-fed lamb-burger-eating graduate school classmates.

When Todd and I broke up a few months later after failing at a long-distance relationship, Keith allayed my fears about losing him as my staple pal in Seattle.

"You're *my* good friend too," he assured me.

I continued to work on getting him a date, broadcasting his many wonderful qualities to my friends.

"He's the greatest guy!" I chimed. "He loves quinoa. He'll make you laugh, he'll ask you questions, and he'll notice when you get a haircut!"

"Why aren't *you* dating him?" they'd ask, as women sometimes do when another single woman sets them up with a male friend.

"He's not my type," I'd say. "It would never work out. Plus, he's my ex-boyfriend's dear friend. Not kosher."

There were no love connections between Keith and my classmates, but I kept at it, even helping to write his profile on the Internet dating site OkCupid. And after enough months passed since my breakup with Todd, I began introducing Keith to the fellows I was dating. I met most of these men on online sites, and we usually didn't make it beyond two or three months. Keith was one of my go-to friends when faith in these fellows faltered, and I was his confidante as he sought advice on the run-ins and telephone exchanges with this elusive species called "women." I rooted for him, and he for me.

"Don't you know some good guys?" I'd lament when another court-ship dissolved after a verbatim "it's not you, it's me" monologue. (I didn't realize those actually happened outside of *My So-Called Life.*)

"Any more cute single girls in your class?" he'd inquire after another walk around the arboretum with an online hookup ended in "That was nice. See you around."

Neither one of us mentioned that when we'd log onto the OkCupid dating site, it consistently matched us up with each other. In bold, it would read on my screen: "Hi, Mary—we show a 94 percent chance that you're a great match for…" and Keith's photo, which I helped him pick out, would flash on the monitor. And I'd press…Delete.

I placated myself with the notion that I barely had time for a relationship anyway. When I wasn't reading, writing, and presenting on studies about the blood pressure-lowering benefits of walnuts or the anti-inflammatory properties of turmeric, I was working as a student clinician at our teaching clinic, seeing patients with a host of medical conditions; volunteering at the local food bank; working as a food server at a hospital; and trying to squeeze in enough yoga to neutralize the hours spent sitting and learning and driving to get to the places where I would sit and learn some more. There was no time for amorous engagement or even a roll in the hay, although I considered that to be a potential cardiac workout that I could justify if I found the right aerobically inclined partner. I directed my affections toward kale (see photo of me with kale), avocados, and buckwheat tortillas, all of which I knew I could rely on as stable companions that rarely disappointed and were always up for a quick picnic.

Beyond Guacamole

What is a rich source of folate, vitamin K, vitamin B, and potassium? Not to mention healthy monounsaturated fats, fiber, and powerful antioxidants? Oh, and have I mentioned the buttery flavor, velvety texture, and rich green color that could inspire Picasso? Throw this all together and you have—yes, you guessed it—the delightfully nutritious avocado! I understood what true foodie love was after biting into a perfectly ripe avocado. The greeting my tongue received from the fleshy meat of this brilliant fruit (yup, it's a fruit!) was like slipping into a down comforter on a brisk day, like biting into fatty silkiness, like munching on what I thought a cloud would feel like when I was six and hadn't yet been taught cloud physics.

Known to be a highly anti-inflammatory food due to its healthy fat content, cholesterol-lowering phytosterols, and diversity of carotenoids (these are plant chemicals with protective antioxidant properties), the avocado has shown benefits for your bones and your ticker. Studies are also now showing potential positive effects on blood sugar and cancer risk. Interestingly enough, the greatest concentration of carotenoids in avocados occurs in the dark green flesh that lies just beneath the skin, so don't fail to scoop out every last piece of avocado "meat."

To those who insist that avocados are fattening (first of all, stop calling my friend names!), I can divulge that half an avocado has approximately 150 calories (less than your average cookie) and offers a low glycemic (a.k.a. low sugar) load with near 12 grams of fat, around 7 grams of fiber, and a touch of protein. Ironically, its high calorie content can actually help with weight loss, since the fat, fiber, and nutrient content help to make your belly feel full, which may prevent additional snacking.

What does one do with this nourishing gem? Avocados are not merely mounds of luscious green guac to top your taco. They can be a creamy alternative to mayo, chopped and thrown into bean and grain salads, served as a replacement to butter in your favorite cookie recipe, or whipped with cocoa powder, maple syrup, and vanilla into a succulent chocolate pudding. Yes, avocado can be a dessert. Wipe that look of disbelief off your face and pop a slice in your mouth before that jaw hits the ground.

An extra tip: Once you have opened an avocado, it's best to store it in a tight container and place in the fridge. Applying a touch of lemon or lime juice will prevent the browning that occurs when it is exposed to oxygen.

References
https://www.ncbi.nlm.nih.gov/pmc/articles/PMC4330060/
https://www.ncbi.nlm.nih.gov/pubmed/8026287
https://www.ncbi.nlm.nih.gov/pubmed/28393409

DORITOS FOR DIABETICS

In order to earn a few bucks and gain some experience in the clinical field during grad school, I decided to become a penguin. I turned into a bird that could not fly. Looks like those acting classes I took in college weren't a waste of time! The gig required my legs to be covered in black polyester that bunched around my hip area, giving me pouches where pouches did not exist. This was matched by an oversized black polyester vest (that hid any hint of breast-like formations) underneath which hung the standard uncreative pleated tuxedo shirt. The top button was sealed not with a bow tie but with a five-dollar plastic circular black clip that shouted, "I may not be as fancy as a bow tie, but I still give this cheap tuxedo an edge of shiny classiness"—and "I'm closing the shirt of someone who could be male or female." I hated this outfit. More than that, I hated the job that required me to wear it.

We were called "dietary ambassadors" of Hillcrest Hospital (not its real name). We were not ambassadors. We were servers. The new food-service manager, inspired by a love of Disney World, called her employees "cast members" (and I didn't even need an agent!) and made sure that all typical food-service nomenclature was gone. And did I mention we looked like penguins?

We stood in the middle of the kitchen at Hillcrest Hospital waiting for the folks assembling the food trays, known as the "food-line expeditors," to yell out, "The meal cart is ready to go to zone 3!" This was all part of a newly implemented system called "room service." All patients had a germ-free and plastic-plated menu in their room to which they could refer in order to procure the dietary delights that they craved after undergoing

19

hip surgery, while in recovery from a gunshot wound, or during treatment for a variety of diseases and ailments that give hospitals their spooky reputation. Once they placed their order, I would write down patients' room numbers as well as the exact minute that they ordered their food so that the time from call to delivery could be tracked and judged.

Once the food was ready, I rolled my assigned cart out of the kitchen and down the hallways of the hospital, where signs plastered every wall declaring this institution as having been voted one of the best places to work in 2004, 2005, and 2006. Photos of well-nourished nurses happily taking the blood pressure of satisfied and photogenic patients lined the corridors. Every time I passed these, I tried to think of what famous person each patient looked like. One was a dead ringer for Dame Judy Dench, except she was wearing a hospital gown and holding an IV line instead of an academy award.

Once in zone 3, I opened up the Velcro-fastened cloth over the cart to reveal the tray destined for room 3705. A special note on the order slip indicated that the patient was a diabetic. Because diabetes means that one's body is less effective at managing sugar in the bloodstream, it would be important for this patient to watch the types of carbohydrates she ate. I peered at the food items on the tray and gasped to myself: diet soda, two chocolate ice creams, and a bag of pretzels. I knew that this was room service but somehow thought the hospital might be invested in seeing her get better (call me a dreamer). Soda, dessert, and high-carb junk food? I could never get that stuff when I was a kid. Who knew that all I had to do was grow up, develop diabetes, and order room service at Hillcrest Hospital?

I knocked on her door. "Room service!" I said like a chirping bellhop ready for a tip.

An agitated voice slathered with weariness responded, "Come in."

I opened the door and beheld a woman whose body was so large that it actually spread across the entire bed like a comforter. Her face was pigeon gray and speckled with sweat beads as she extended her hand to receive the bounty of sugar I was delivering. I appeased my discomfort with the thought, "The hospital dietitians must know what they are doing."

"Enjoy your meal," I mumbled, wincing at my word choice. I should have said, "Enjoy your strychnine! Have fun chewing on that Agent Orange! God bless."

As I made my way to the next room, I avoided thinking about the crime it felt like I had just committed. I tried to make small talk with a fellow dietary ambassador in training who was shadowing me for the day. That's right: I was her personal guide on how to speed up the demise of patients at Hillcrest Hospital. She also worked as a hairdresser and sported several fiery flashes of orange in her straight long black hair. I didn't mention the poisoning episode, as I wasn't yet convinced as to whether her allegiance lay with the hospital or with common sense. I handed her a tray of food for room 3709 (a female stroke patient) replete with all the things that a stroke victim might need: a cheeseburger with chips, a chocolate brownie, and a high caffeine soda. I almost had a stroke looking at this "meal," but my trainee didn't seem to notice the potential relationship between the contents on the tray and the status of the specimen in room 3709. And yes! The time from order to delivery: fourteen minutes. A success according to our food service manager, or shall I say, "effective nutrition delivery designer."

When she returned, I made no comments. Instead, I inquired about her salon, mused about hair products, asked her to describe her styling specialties—anything to take my mind off of the blood clot that would soon be forming in room 3709's leg. I realized that after four minutes, there was nothing left to talk about. We stood side by side rolling the cart of doom down the hall in complete and total silence. I thought hairstylists were adept in the art of small talk and meaningless banter, but apparently she was either stunned into silence or had missed the training on chitchat. I couldn't think of a single thing to say beyond screaming, "I just gave two ice creams and a bag of Rold Gold pretzels to a morbidly obese diabetic woman with necrotic feet!" My conversation skills were experiencing their own necrosis.

Back at the kitchen, we prepared more trays of deliciously nutritious food created by the cooks (a.k.a. "nourishment architects"). I loaded a "heart-healthy" meal onto my cart for zone 2: fish and chips, a Rice

Krispies treat, and a lemon lime soda. Yes, this dish was actually starred as "heart-healthy." The inferior vena cava was going to be thrilled.

"We need more vanilla pudding and chocolate milk," bellowed one of the expeditors busily setting up four trays of heart-attack stew and stroke casserole. This was not what I signed up for when I applied for a job to gain experience in the food-management arena for my master's degree in clinical nutrition. Instead of being a purveyor of health and healing, I was more like an accomplice in a murder plot for the sick. It felt like a mafia movie where the least likely suspect suddenly start killing off the weak. I looked around to see if maybe I had walked into a Red Robin restaurant or an Applebee's instead of a hospital where people came to get *well.* Nope, it was Hillcrest all right. I was still in my tuxedo—stained with low-sodium tartar sauce from the fish and chips plate—and surrounded by my fellow flightless birds who seemed to have no awareness of the edible booby traps they were arranging.

Jeremy (not his real name), the head nourishment architect—a very large man whose torso sloped down on a diagonal, ending at his protruding belly—asked me why I was standing around not doing anything. "I'm waiting for more trays of your terrific food to be ready," I muttered weakly. I wondered if he was able to discern the anti-establishment sentiments in my speech pattern or intuit my plan for a hospital mutiny. I had fantasized about opening the food drawers and walk-in freezer and tossing out the trans-fat-filled strawberry shortcake and bacon, ditching the high-sodium Doritos and Cheetos, and opening up packages of frozen berries and broccoli as if they were all caged birds trapped at a pet store. Instead, I busied myself by scooting over to the soda machine to attend to the worthwhile task of making certain that the Diet Pepsi spout wasn't mistakenly spewing out Dr. Pepper.

Thirteen dollars an hour. Was it worth the moral angst? I thought about the sample menu that I helped to design in my therapeutic cooking class at school for "Bob," my mock patient, who had food allergies and digestive distress, not to mention a busy schedule. We had given him a healing miso soup with napa cabbage, daikon radish, carrots, onions, organic turkey, and aduki beans as well as a spectrum of nutrient-dense side dishes to help him on his journey to wellness. I bet that Head Nourishment Architect, Jeremy, probably wouldn't even know what to do with aduki beans. I imagined the kitchen staff's response to my suggestion of Bob's menu for some of the patients here.

"Gross."

"Huh?"

"What the hell is napa cabbage?"

What is napa cabbage, indeed! Why would anyone want that when there are Danishes and donuts for Auntie Sue's breakfast, Philly cheese steak for Grandpa's lunch, and gravy-smothered pork loin for your sick mama's dinner?

But I needed this job and I didn't feel like being a rabble-rouser that day. I had already sparked a heated debate when I suggested that the artificial sweetener aspartame was potentially risky. Hell, Hillcrest probably bathed their patients in aspartame. It was perhaps what was flowing through their IV lines. Poor Dame Judy Dench look-alike lady!

I decided to save my rebellion for another day. I loaded another tray onto my cart—cream of cancer soup with a side of hypertension going to zone 1—and slowly exited the kitchen carrying what felt like a scythe and an executioner's mask.

What to Do with Aduki Beans*

First of all, just saying the word *aduki* is fun. Say it aloud! "Aduki." Your mouth has to form a smile with that third syllable allowing this bean to have health-promoting properties just in the simple recitation of its handle. (Please note: it is sometimes referred to as the "adzuki" bean. Choose your favorite version. Saying "zzzzz" is also lingually entertaining so that may be your preference.)

These edible nuggets are popular in Chinese and Japanese cuisine. In fact, if you have ever enjoyed the red-bean paste in a bun or mochi ball, you may have munched on adzukis without even knowing it. These reddish beans are usually mixed with sugar to create those yummy innards, but they're equally scrumptious as a savory meal and can be substituted for anything you might make with black beans.

I cannot compliment these beans (or "pulses," as they are calling them now) enough for their health-promoting prowess. Are you ready for impressive nutrition stats? One cup of adzukis has around 16 grams of plant-based protein,(approximately one-quarter of a typical person's needs), 16 grams of fiber (around half of the recommended daily recommended amount, although I recommend about three times that much) and provide you with excellent sources of vitamins and minerals like folate, potassium, and magnesium, sufficient amounts of which just make you a healthier human (and perhaps a better person?). Plus, that reddish color I was referring to (call it crimson, scarlet, or cranberry if you like) usually means there are plant chemicals present. These are good and naturally occurring chemicals, unlike Windex or paint thinner, which can exert a protective effect. What's not to love so far?

What about taste? These little *pulsitos* (my pet name) have a nutty flavor which pairs well with veggies and goes great in a hearty stew. They are often the bean that makes up the protein

---

* See the *Mary's Nutrition Show* episode "Live to be 100: A Nutritional Hill of Beans": https://youtu.be/Rk8p55A7-tQ

portion of a macrobiotic bowl, a very simple style of eating with a focus on beans, grains, and veggies, usually slathered in tahini sauce. Like many beans, it may be the herbs, spices, and sauces you use that makes the difference in the flavor of the meal. Love coconut curry? Add that to your preparation efforts. Adore onions? Well, introduce the two and let the magic happen!

Good news: if you are concerned about heart disease or diabetes or obesity, beans have been shown in "the literature" (that's the vast amount of research out there that has been scientifically validated, not a collection of scenes from Dickens, Charlotte Brontë, or Toni Morrison) to aid in the prevention of these chronic medical conditions. So go grab a can of adzukis (yes, it's ok to eat canned beans, just eat them, for crying out loud! http://www.edenfoods.com/store/aduki-beans-organic-bpa-free-lined-can.html) or buy some dried beans in bulk, soak overnight, and then cook them up (this is ok too, if you have the time; I'm mostly a canned-beans chick, myself.)

All in favor of branching out into the bean world starting with adzukis say "aye." Aye!

I love this recipe for Adzuki and Yam Hash from one of my favorite go-to cookbooks, Nourishing Meals, by Tom Malterre and Alyssa Segersten. www.nourishingmeals.com.

Mary Purdy, MS, RDN

Adzuki Bean and Yam Hash

As long as you have your adzuki beans cooked and a pot of quinoa on the stove, you'll be able to whip this recipe up in no time. The key is to dice the yams very small; that way, they cook quickly without burning.

2 tablespoons extra virgin olive oil
1 medium onion, diced
2 medium yams, peeled and diced small
2 teaspoons dried thyme
1/2 to 1 teaspoon ground cumin
2 cups cooked adzuki beans
4 to 5 collard greens, finely chopped*

Herbamare and black pepper to taste

Heat a large skillet over medium heat. I use an 11-inch stainless-steel skillet. Add olive oil, onion, and a few dashes of salt. Sauté for a few minutes.

Then add yams, thyme, and cumin. Sauté for a few minutes uncovered, then cover your pan and cook for about 15 to 20 minutes, stirring occasionally, until yams are tender. Watch carefully so they don't burn.

Add adzuki beans and collard greens. Sauté a few minutes more or until collards are tender. Add Herbamare and pepper to taste.

*Note: To finely chop collard greens, first stack the leaves on top of each other. Then tightly roll. Use a sharp knife to thinly slice the collards, then cut those slices crosswise into small pieces.

Source: http://www.nourishingmeals.com/2010/01/adzuki-bean-yam-hash.html

References

https://www.ncbi.nlm.nih.gov/pubmed/24710915
https://www.ncbi.nlm.nih.gov/pubmed/25061763
https://www.ncbi.nlm.nih.gov/pubmed/24710915

GUM BAN IN THE PURDY HOUSEHOLD; OR, WHY I DON'T CHEW GUM

Just why am I so crazy about adzuki beans and so horrified by Cheetos? Well, it could have all started with Bubble Yum. Or rather, my mom's ban on it.

The Purdy household was more likely to be found eating salads than Stouffer's and sitting around a table actually talking. This is saying something, seeing as it was the '70s, the era of Velveeta, Twinkies, and conversation-stopping TV dinners. We were allowed one "semijunk" cereal per month. Froot Loops, Cap'n Crunch, and Lucky Charms were absolutely forbidden, so my older brother and I decided ours would be Honey Comb cereal. (It is possible that my somewhat tyrannical older brother, Chris, may have made this decision for us, as I was pretty much his dutiful and rule-following minion for my entire childhood.) I was also totally fixated on pretty much all confections. However, any purchase of Oreo cookies had to come out of our own allowance money. Fig Newtons were acceptable. Nutter Butters were not. Neither was bubble gum. According to my mother, it was hideous for a variety of reasons.

Dear Children,

This notice is to announce that gum has been officially banned in our household. Why? First off, you look terrible when you chew it—like a cow, like a cheap street walker, like someone who has no manners and uses improper grammar.

Secondly, it gives off the unpleasant odor of artificial junk. Doublemint gum is the exception here, but we'll address the problems with that momentarily. Bubble Yum, Dubble Bubble, and Bazooka are never to be mentioned to me. Their sickly sweet ersatz scent is enough to make me tear my dissertation out of the typewriter and grab that steaming saliva-ridden ball of crap out of your mouth and throw it all in the garbage. Did you hear me? I am writing my dissertation on a *typewriter.* That means it isn't saved, and if the popping and smacking forces me to rip it up, I'd have to write it all over again. You don't want me to do that, do you?

I am digressing here, but I feel pretty strongly about this, so I'm just going with it.

Reason #3. Wait. Did I cover #2? Ah, yes, the toxic cherry smell of that pink blob of nothing that I see hiding out between your teeth.

#3: Someone went to bed chewing their Doublemint gum (that person will remain nameless for now), and we all know how badly that turns out. Here's where I get to lambast Wrigley's Doublemint. While it has a fairly tolerable scent, Doublemint gum is a lot thinner than Dubble Bubble or Bubble Yum and therefore has a tendency to stick more readily to surfaces, which, *Mary Purdy,* is exactly what it did to your pillowcases after you decided to go to bed with it *still in your mouth.* Did you honestly think it would stay there for eight hours? So while you were doubling your pleasure, I was doubling my workload in the washer. Have I mentioned I am working on my PhD? I don't have time for extra work like extracting dried gum pieces from linens. I am trying to do something important!

Finally, I'm not sure if you've perused the health section of the *New York Times,* but sugary gum causes cavities. Yes, cavities! (Remember that it is still 1978 and we haven't realized that sugar also increases the risk of diabetes, which will essentially bankrupt our health-care economy, but I cannot ponder the future right now. I have a dissertation and gummy linens to worry about!) Cavities are little brown holes in your teeth that your father and I have to pay money to have a humorless dentist with a pronounced butt-like cleft in his chin, fill up with little tufts of silver mercury, which are probably even more toxic than Bubble Yum.* This is not something that you enjoy, and it certainly isn't something that we enjoy paying for, so let's lessen the burden on all of us in the household and keep it as far away from the apartment as possible.

Please do not attempt to hide that gummy gob under your tongue. I can tell from your garbled sentences that it is lodged there, and remember that I have the nose of a bloodhound.

Thank you for your attention to this matter.

Your Mom**

---

* I actually chewed something similar to Bubble Yum recently, and I totally agree with my mom that it is, in fact, completely toxic and disgusting. Why are moms always right?
** See the *Mary's Nutrition Show* episode "5 Things to Help Sugar Cravings": https://youtu.be/POmFa2PbqlA.

THE SMELL OF DONUTS STILL MAKES ME WEEP

I am not normally prone to weeping. I'll sniffle occasionally at a Meryl Streep movie or an old episode of *Emergency Vets*. You might hear me choke up in an attempt to speak about a loved one at some ceremonious occasion. But one does not generally find me in a crumpled ball surrounded by a flood of salty tears. Until…I decided to buy a new car.

Inspired by my Seattle surroundings and my "Sustainable Food Systems" course, I was seriously going green. Even with my social justice and hippie leanings, environmental preservation hadn't made it to my top-ten priority list when I was living in New York City. I was a lazy recycler (five cents per bottle? Meh…), nor did I even consider the impact I might be having when I dumped the leftover moldy chicken with broccoli from my fridge into the trash. I saw it as garbage that needed to be disposed of. But in Seattle, eco-living was a religion. The lunch room at Bastyr University (my graduate school) had a spot for composting and a special bucket dedicated to recycling batteries. All coffee shops gave you a discount when you brought your own mug. The city sent out large trucks to your home weekly to pick up your yard waste and bring it to its new home, the delightfully titled "Cedar Grove Compost" (the best graveyard name ever).

I ate and shopped local, dined at organic/farm-to-table restaurants, and finished whatever I put on my plate. What I didn't eat got transferred into a compostable receptacle and delivered to the leftovers section of my fridge. I was also known to finish or take home what was left on other people's plates. I know, this may sound a little icky, but I couldn't bear to see it get tossed and was undeterred by what I felt as the "myth of germs." (Please see my final essay about a very unsanitary act I performed as a toddler and still lived to tell the tale.) I avoided food packaging and carried around a tea tumbler for every liquid I planned to consume. I purchased recycled toilet paper; selected environmentally friendly dish-washing, clothes-washing, face-cleansing (good-bye, beloved Noxzema!), body-scrubbing, and counter-cleaning products; and started compost-ing...everything, including the hair from my hairbrush. I flushed only when necessary and forwent one shower each week on minimal-sweating days when I had no plans for any exceptionally close hugging.

Most of what I owned—clothes, furniture, electronics, pots, pans, mugs, forks, and spoons—had originally been, in their newness, in the hands of someone else. As I began to scan the larger contributors to my carbon footprint, I saw potential further eco-salvation in the purchase of an alternative car that relied not on Chevron but on the transformed substance from the discards of the local greasy spoon: biodiesel. My friends, Keith and Andy, each had biodiesel cars, and I had not heard a negative peep about unusual car trouble or fuel access. Biodiesel sta-tions were popping up in a few nearby neighborhoods, and I had caught word of a couple of guys who made their own stuff from discarded tem-pura batter. Keith was a customer, and despite my nutritionist-in-training status, I enjoyed the subtle sweet scent of donuts when riding in his rig.

"Plus," Keith told me, "you get more miles to the gallon, and you don't feel guilty when you idle in traffic."

"Yes," I thought. "This is, indeed, the right next step for my con-science and my wallet."

My fifteen-year-old Buick was not easy on the environment, oil fields, or eyes for that matter. The dried-up SPF 15 lotion I had accidentally spilled across the entire dashboard two years prior during my drive out to Seattle from New York City had stained the area, likening it to a lame Jackson Pollack painting. I had neglected to clean it for months, think-ing that when I "had the time" (i.e. the seven minutes it might take to bring a washcloth and Windex out to the car), I'd get to it. But there was always either an exam on riboflavin and folate to study for or a paper on "The Benefits of Seaweed" to be written, or another lame online date to unnecessarily shave my legs for, so those seven minutes never appeared, and I was now stuck with a permanently sullied console. Plus, I was becoming weary of having to manually click my left turn signal, which had refused to work on its own accord over the past year, eliciting many curious looks and comments from those in the passenger seat about why I was fondling my automobile every time I needed to make a left turn.

After a test drive with a biodiesel Mercedes left me feeling as if I was behind the wheel of a large sailing vessel, I determined to sleuth out a daintier model. I searched the Internet for one that I hoped would elevate me to the position of official snubber of Exxon and his evil siblings, Shell and Arco. Adding to my eagerness for a speedy purchase was an impending five-hour drive to a snowy section of Oregon for a solo holiday retreat that would require the use of a more trustworthy vehicle than my Buick, which sputtered, stammered, and slid in any hint of precipitation.

One late evening, after overdosing on fats, carbs, and protein (textbook readings, that is!), I decided to "surf the net." (Do people still call it that? Did they ever call it that for more than the seven minutes it might have taken to clean my dashboard?) I happened upon an ad on Craigslist for biodiesel cars that could be shipped by an individual vendor from Montana. One cute and hip VW Golf was right in my price range. I write "VW Golf" as if I actually knew what that even meant at the time. Hailing from New York City, where I didn't get a license until I was twenty-five years old, I had a brief moment when I thought the listing might be referring to a golf cart.

Luckily, a conversation with the seller, "Scott," cleared that up, and I began to move forward with the purchasing proceedings. There were references given and phone calls made to former customers with glowing reviews of this car peddler, followed by a friendly phone conversation with "John," an affable auto mechanic in Montana who checked out the Golf and gave it the oil-stained thumbs-up. It was all clear. I felt ready to complete the wire transfer and join the ranks of French-fry-scented exhaust-pipe proprietors. The car would arrive two days before my trip to snowy Oregon, and I would be all set to go. In my excitement, I called my friend, Andy, my fellow biodiesel enthusiast, to share my eco-news.

"That's great," he said. "Is it an automatic or a stick shift?"

Mary Purdy, MS, RDN

I chuckled. "Oh, it's an automatic, of course. I don't know how to drive a stick shift." The organic apple slice I had just eaten backed up into my throat. *Was* it an automatic? Had Scott and I discussed that? Did John make mention of it as he enumerated the many aspects about the car that were functional?

"Uh, Scott," I asked over the phone that evening, "This is a silly question, but the car isn't a *stick* shift, is it?"

"It sure is," Scott said cheerily. "That's what it said in the ad: 'five-speed.'"

My lower lip dangled. Rhubarb crisp churned in my stomach. Five-speed. Yes, I remembered seeing that. However, in my vehicular ignorance, I had thought, "Sure, five-speed. Sounds great. That's what cars do. They have speeds. Really slow, slow, kind of fast, fast, superfast." Shit.

The wire transfer for thousands of dollars of my money (or Gramma's money, which she left for me when she died—thanks, Gramma!) was in progress as I drooled in disbelief on the phone mouthpiece.

"Uh, Scott," I faltered. "I don't know how to drive a stick shift. I'm not a strong driver on an automatic. I'm not sure I even know what having a stick shift means."

A long exhale emerged from the end of the line. "Well, it *was* in the ad, Mary." His voice lilted upward like a dad trying to look on the bright side of a dropped ice-cream cone. "In any case, stick shifts are more fun. They make you feel like you are actually doing the driving because *you're* more in control."

I didn't want to be in control. I just wanted to sit down and put my gear into drive until I stopped and needed to put it into park. I didn't need to have fun while I drove. I just wanted to get to my "Food Science" class, my internship at the Kidney Dialysis Center, the organic grocery store, or to a visit with friends who lived further than a bike or bus ride away. I had visions of trying to be in control of five speeds on top of a snowbank on my five-hour drive to Oregon. Curse my foolishly blind aspirations to be green.

"Let me let this all sink in, ok, Scott?" I said. "I'm going to make a few phone calls, maybe meditate on this for a minute, and I'll call you back."

We hung up, and I immediately telephoned Keith, whose donut-mobile was also a stick shift, but he was fortunately (for him) out of town. Of course, his first response was, "You bought a biodiesel car! That's great! Now Joanie [the name of his biodiesel car] has a friend." He was the one who had sent me the "Seattle Yard Waste" link months earlier and gently informed me that the toilet-paper roll in my garbage can belonged with its soon-to-be-reborn pieces of paper in the recycling bin. I knew he'd be a fan.

"What good is it if I can't drive it?" I moaned.

"You're gonna be awesome," he said. "I'll hook you up with my black-market Bio-D source when I get back."

Next, I called three stick-shift-owning friends, explaining in verbal burps: "Internet...Montana...five-speed...Scott...John...biodiesel...killing the environment." In fifteen minutes, I had three lessons set up and a healthy meditated-upon vision of me driving happily "in full control" to Oregon, shifting away, my smile swelling with each gear. I called Scott.

"It's a go!" I said, oozing forced ebullience in my tenuous car confidence.

With the Golf due to arrive on Thursday evening, I had scheduled lessons on Monday and Tuesday to give me ample time to prepare my right hand and left foot for the additional jerking and thrusting I presumed was necessary to operate a standard.

However, the stick-shift tutorials left me more insecure than I was in my original moment of panic after learning the true nature of my vehicle. My patient instructors, who also agreed to let me practice on their cars, attempted to soothe my nervous energy.

"You're doing great," encouraged my pal Andy as I stalled in the middle of a driving island, a toothless ruffian in a yellow truck honking madly behind us.

"Ease up on the clutch," advised Pete, my second teacher, as my left foot disengaged, sending us both shooting forward into the grasp of our seat belts, the car no longer running.

I hated the clutch. I hated the stick shift. I hated the environment for being so susceptible to ruin by my comforting twenty-miles-a-gallon Buick. I quickly whipped up and stress-ate a "pecan date bonbon" ball, and when that didn't help, I ripped open a bar of non-fair-trade chocolate and didn't recycle the packaging.

Two girlfriends, Vanessa and Kris, gave me my final lesson on the terrifying downtown streets of Seattle, pelleting me with the advice "Neutral is your friend" and something along the lines of "You can roll into second gear," a suggestion I would need later that night but which I promptly forgot as soon as I stepped out of the car and onto solid ground, my left leg still buzzing from the exerted pressure.

When the new Golf finally trundled into my driveway late Thursday night, delivered by two lovely Polish fellows who spoke not a lick of English, I thought I'd give it a go on my own. With the late hour, I figured there'd be less light to reveal my lack of license plates and fewer people into whom I might crash. I hopped into the driver's seat, revved up the engine, eased into reverse, and slowly but successfully backed out of my driveway onto a road heading west.

As I was basking in the surprising glow of confidence at having mastered my new vehicle, I noticed that many cars were seemingly coming out of nowhere and heading toward me, awaiting my next move. At first the drivers idled patiently behind me while I cautiously switched from reverse into first gear, released gently my left foot while pushing gently (*gently!* Andy and Pete had warned!) with my right and...kaphlumph, the VW halted. *I was four feet out of my driveway.* Ignition started, deep breath, determination in my soul, left foot on the clutch ready to release, right foot on the gas ready to give and...kaphlumph. Repeat. Kaphlumph. Repeat. Kaphlumph.

There I sat in the middle of the road, stalled just minutes after my initial and triumphant exit from my driveway. I began to roll backward down the street. Little liquid beads started dripping down my lower back, which only happens after I've been in the sauna for fifteen minutes or when I sense potential harm in the immediate future. Cars started to slowly pass me, their drivers glancing sideways at me. A large grapefruit formed in the back of my throat. I rolled down my window and waved them forward, hoping my twiggy wrist and tightly knuckled hand didn't reveal my truth as an inexpert car wussy.

Who buys a car without seeing it and knowing she is without the skill-set to drive it? The grapefruit turned to a small unripe cantaloupe as I crept out of the VW and stood there mouthing "I'm sorry!" to the oncoming cars, signaling them to pass this metal lump in the road. Finally, a guy not more than seventeen stopped (perhaps noticing my trembling lower lip) and offered to at least get me off the slanting road and onto more leveled ground. I readily accepted, and minutes later, with the car still purring, I was back in the driver's seat having gotten the thumbs-up from this kind whippersnapper for my eco-wheels. As I was mustering up my confidence to try again, it dawned on me that I was in Seattle, where hills make up most of the terrain. I imagined the audience members watching the movie of my life screaming "Don't do it! Get *out* of the car!" Ignoring my intuition, I turned on the ignition.

First gear, and I was inching my way back onto the street. Second gear, and I made a right turn. Third gear, and it felt like the car was trying to drive itself. Ok, I told myself. Slow down. This was a residential neighborhood where there were small children and curious cats. Ten worrisome minutes and seven blocks later, I was gripping the steering wheel so hard, I looked like I had scleroderma, the autoimmune joint disease I had just seen a presentation on months earlier in school. (It ain't pretty, believe me.)

It was dark. I was on a steep one-way street that I had turned onto by mistake. I was rolling backward and not in any way, shape, or form "in control" of my vehicle by any DMV or Scott the VW salesman standards. Those beads of liquid had made their way down to my butt crack and were forming a small pool. The fruit in the back of my throat had become a sizeable watermelon. Brake.

The blubbering began, deep and throaty. I mustered up enough tears to wipe clean the dashboard of my old Buick. It wasn't just the car debacle. It was everything: "I hate working at the hospital. I'm sick of being single. I'm not as close with my brother as I want to be. I can't stop grinding my teeth at night. I'm messy. I have no health care. My friends are different since they had kids. I worry about my Dad. I don't know what I'm going to do with a nutrition degree. I'll never find that hand-knit sweater from my grandma that I left on the bus. Injustice prevails in the world." (Normally, I wouldn't put these last two on equal footing, but when you're upset and feeling inadequate, lost sweater = injustice.)

It was as if my car headlights were suddenly spotlighting all my flaws and life's foibles. The sobbing weakened my grip on the clutch, and I could feel the car rolling backward once again. This time, it was the emergency brake I yanked up. No more chances. I pulled out and flipped open my cell phone (yes, the recycled one that might as well have been a rotary) and called Andy, my friend most likely to be awake and whom I hoped could calmly guide me through driving down a hill in reverse in the glow of a weak lamppost. He answered, and my voice choked.

"Andy, I'm in the VW Golf rolling backward down a fucking hill on the corner of 45th and 2nd Avenue."

He talked me down. Literally. Inch by inch, I made my way backward down the street in neutral—which, it turned out, *was* my friend. I made it home, mascara-stained cheeks and all. and hobbled inside my house to shower my soaked backside and relive the entire episode as I slept.

The next day, I called Avis and rented a four-wheel drive Subaru for the five-hour trip to Oregon. Best decision ever, considering the four-foot-high snow bank I had to back out of to start my trip home.

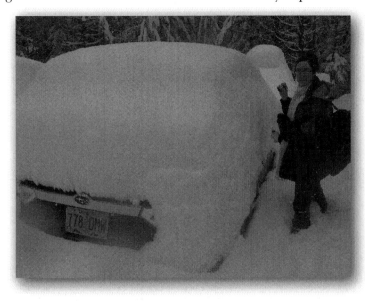

Eventually I learned to drive the Golf and came to feel that the stick shift was kind of like having my own penis that I could knock around whenever I wanted to. I became known at the various clinical rotations of my dietetic internship not as the woman who brought donuts into the office (c'mon, I brought in kale chips!) but the woman who brought the *smell* of donuts into the parking garage. I'd call Keith's underground bio-diesel dudes (a.k.a. "the boys") claiming myself as a "friend of Keith"— magic words that garnered me four-dollars-a-gallon fry oil from the secret greasy-clump-swathed garage and a fifteen-minute conversation about Elon Musk, the EPA, and the sundry uses for coffee grounds. I continued the determination to bring my carbon footprint down from Sasquatch size to that of Cinderella's dainty slipper, even in small ways like using my Golf to transport household and closet castoffs to Goodwill instead of the dump; hopping at farmers' markets with my seven canvas bags; and, yes, reusing dental floss (my own, of course), because it is actually pretty much tough enough for a few flossings! The tears and fears that accompanied my foray into the five-speed car adventure fortified and wizened me in several ways: #1. Read the fine print, or rather, *look up the definition of* the print itself, Mary Purdy, so you know what you are getting into. #2. Being a steward of the earth doesn't require you to be perfect. (Sometimes I threw my banana peel into the garbage by mistake. Apologies, Mother Nature!) #3. (This one's a bit more metaphorical. Just go with it.) While, yes, I can roll easily into second gear, it's super important not to get stuck there. Sometimes it takes the support of friends, kind strangers and a guy named Scott from Montana to help get to third. And for that, I am grateful.

Eco-Eating Tips; or, How to Go Green without Rolling Backward down a Hill in a Car You Cannot Drive*

Feel free to check these off as you go along.

1. **Eat more vegetarian more often**. ☐ (Friendly note: This is not a directive around becoming vegan, so no need to start hollering about giving up bacon.) Here's the skinny: Meat production is responsible for 13 percent of our greenhouse gases. These gases come from the methane produced by the digestive tracts of our animals—yes, I'm talking about the unprecedented amount of flatulence that occurs when cows eat a trough of grains. Additionally, it takes two thousand gallons of water to produce one pound of beef. (One pound of beef = about four regular sized hamburger patties.) One pound of grains or tofu use about three hundred gallons of water—still quite a bit but alarmingly less. Interesting fact: one pound of cricket flour takes one gallon of water. I know that you may think of crickets as chirping in fields and not crackling in a pan, but these little guys are edible. While this is not technically vegetarian and perhaps frightfully offensive to Jiminy Cricket fans, it may be something you start hearing more about as a sustainable food source. Meat production also takes up a lot of land—both as a place for animals to hang out as well as the space used to grow the grains that make these bovines so unpleasant to have as guests at your dinner party.

   If everyone in the United States ate vegetarian once a week, it would be the equivalent of taking around half a million cars off the road. Are you craving that cup of lentil soup yet?

   Reference: http://www.ewg.org/meateatersguide/a-meat-eaters-guide-to-climate-change-health-what-you-eat-matters/reducing-your-footprint/

---

* See the *Mary's Nutrition Show* episode "Eat Sustainably: Mary's Climate Accord": https://youtu.be/R8zn0LumWm8.

2. **Reduce food waste.** ☐ We throw away a third of the food that we produce. It breaks my heart to even write this, because that is utterly absurd and unnecessary. This means that the typical American wastes 1,300 calories every day—enough for a person to have close to a day's worth of meals. If you are interested in what that could look like, here is an example: Blueberry Oatmeal from Starbucks = 220 cals + Tuna Sammy from Subway = 470 cals + 1 oz almonds from Trader Joe's = 160 cals + ½ Chipotle Veggie Burrito = 420 cals. Add that all together and you've got 1,270 calories. You've got 30 calories to spare. Well, heck! Let's add in 1 cup of broccoli, because you didn't get many veggies in all that. One cup of broccoli = 30 cals. Done—1,300 cals. Can you imagine the hungry tummies swirling with gratitude for those vittles?

    The wasted food that sits in landfills produces more methane gas, which contributes to our greenhouse gases. Let us be clear (like the politicians like to say): this is not about being a member of the clean-plate club and forcing yourself to scarf down food you don't need just for the sake of not wasting. I do not advise this. But there are many ways to avoid throwing away food in the first place.

    -   **Order less when you eat out!** ☐ Or take home your leftovers for a meal the next day. Extra bonus: bring your own container with you so you aren't using one of theirs.
    -   **Clean out your refrigerator!** ☐ It's probably time anyway, and you may discover a treasure that you forgot you had. Give that flaccid carrot in the back there a chance to be thrown into a hearty soup before it becomes a science experiment. Full disclosure: I recently allowed an entire tub of applesauce to ferment and become alcoholic (not in a good way) after neglecting to make those apple muffins I promised my husband I'd make when I initially opened the jar. I have apologized to Mother Nature for this transgression and will do my best to avoid a repeat.

3. **Don't overlook the aesthetically challenged foods at the grocery store or your farmers market.** □ All foods are beautiful, despite what your eight-year-old daughter/son/nephew/ niece/random child at the grocery store says. A couple months back, I bought a daikon radish that looked like a small person in a straightjacket (see photo here), but it tasted just as delicious as the pristine version I had purchased the week earlier. Plus, my husband had a field day taking photos. So, grab that goofy-looking piece of fruit and the malformed vegetable and turn off the voice in your head that says that apples must be perfectly round and that carrots weren't meant to have arms.

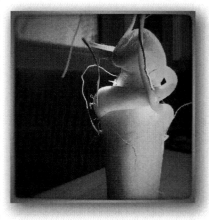

4. **Use less packaging/buy in bulk!** □ I know this is hard, especially when there is an enticing and perfectly symmetrical photo of a bowl of coconut flax seed granola on the box or a heartwarming logo of an older man who could be a family member on your rice package. The bulk section (that area where you scoop nuts, grains, dried fruit, and cereals into an unadorned baggie) is usually more affordable and allows for fewer resources to be used in our food production. "But I love my poblano black-bean burger that I buy from the freezer section," you say. (Me too!) That's fine. Buy it and eat it and love it. (And thank you for eating a vegetarian burger. Please check the box next to Tip #1.) But for nature's sake, recycle the damn box. Don't throw it in the garbage. Get thee over to the garbage and let it know it has been "reassigned" to the recycling bin. No recycling? Call your local city council (https://www.usa. gov/local-governments) and welcome them to 2018.

UNEXPECTED SOMERSAULTS OF THE HEART

Two years after the cherries and popcorn-movie outings with my friend Keith, my subconscious started playing tricks on me. I woke up one morning with a funny feeling that I had been naked with someone...Keith? Yes! I dreamed I was naked with and kissing Keith. "That's odd. I'm not attracted to him," I told myself. "We are just friends or... like cousins even!" It didn't matter that we loved spending time together, always made each other laugh, enjoyed the same activities, supported and were always there to lend an ear in times of trouble. It was *inappropriate*. He was my ex's cherished buddy from grad school.

I pushed it out of my flustered head and told no one. I told *myself* that I didn't have enough time, energy, or bandwidth for something with this kind of potential (to succeed or fail). I could foresee things being completely awkward and embarrassing, feelings getting hurt, and our friendship being obliterated. Anyway, I was in the midst of the rigorous and time-consuming dietetic internship of my nutrition graduate program and was done navigating through complex chemical reactions.

But when he and I went salsa dancing one night, my heart started somersaulting as we tore across the dance floor pretending to be Latin lovers whispering fake romantic Spanish words as we stared into each other's eyes. I panicked. What was happening? I was not supposed to be feeling things for someone I had started considering a close family member and whose history with my ex-boyfriend, Todd, had the potential to turn this into an episode of *Grey's Anatomy* or the next Ric Ocasek song.

I'd never been this close to a male who wasn't a romantic partner, and it was messing with my well-ingrained perception of what friendship could be and what partnership should be. Confused and unnerved by this disorder in my heart and mind, I immediately began to date the tallest, skinniest, un-Keith-like guy I could find. He smoked, regularly ate at Jack in the Box, and was not even remotely allergic to soy. After this silly escapade of poor judgment ended a couple months later—I could not be with someone who electively consumed trans fats and inhaled sticks of cancer*—Keith's face and body started showing up again in my mind, but this time while I was awake.

I was working more than forty hours a week at a variety of community and clinical settings and having trouble focusing. Was I looking for an excuse to drift away from the monotony of school meal planning and low potassium renal diets,** or was the Keith fantasia the real deal? I consulted a mutual friend of ours, swearing her to secrecy.

"I think I'm having *those* feelings," I reported cautiously, whispering out of the side of my mouth so the strangers next to us wouldn't suspect anything. Her elated response led me to believe that maybe I wasn't a total crazy lady.

"It's about time," she said, shaking her head and rolling her eyes to the heavens.

When Keith left for a monthlong silent retreat, I began to miss him, think about him, and, gulp…read his horoscope. I called and left messages on his voicemail "just to say hi" and hoped he was having a "great time being all silent and stuff." When he returned, he told me that when he checked his phone at the end of his four-week retreat, there were three messages. All from me.

"I just wanted to make sure I didn't forget to tell you a few things when you got back," I fibbed.

---

* I also spent Thanksgiving with him and his mother and gagged on, I mean, feasted on slimy canned green beans, tasteless stovetop stuffing soaked in I Can't Believe It's Not Butter, soggy corn, and toxic orange Jell-O.

** Renal diets are for people who have compromised kidney function; their kidneys don't filter out potassium as well as mine or yours do. (Unless you have kidney issues. Do you have kidney issues? If so, I can help design a healthy low-potassium diet for you. I assure you, I was paying attention despite my Keith-infused wandering mind.)

A few days after he returned, we planned to meet at a mutual friend's party. When I walked in the door, he was in a corner chatting with someone with a glass of red wine in one hand. He had grown a goatee. (Please see one of my earlier essays where I mention how I feel about facial hair. I'm *wild* about goatees.) He was wearing a blue turtleneck. Turtlenecks on men drive me wild. (I didn't mention this in any of my previous essays, but I assure you, it's true, and I plan to dedicate at least a sentence if not an entire paragraph to this in my next book.) He was smiling and laughing (and probably listening and asking questions and noticing that person's haircut and...). "Oh, God," I thought and swallowed hard as I approached, hugged him, and smiled casually, trying to conceal my skipping heartbeat and weak bladder.

I stood there trying to listen to him speak and not nuzzle my head between his beard and turtleneck. I thought I could just very simply let him know my feelings, in a fun, no-pressure, no-big-deal, *well, whaddya think about that?* kind of way. The thought of losing him as a friend was terrifying, but the phrase "I think I *like you,* like you" was ready to leap off my tongue. Yet baring my soul at a cocktail party while '80s music blared in the background and acquaintances weaved in and out of our circle just didn't fit my vision of the romantic reveal, so I pressed pause on my plan. I needed to see if my heart palpitations and compromised bladder control at the sight of him was just a one-time fluke. Maybe it was just all that green tea I was consuming.

When we went out for dinner at a Middle Eastern joint the following week, my physiological response to my Keith crush moved from bladder to belly. As munchkins danced about with pitchforks inside my internal organs, I tried not to become overly giddy as he squirted Karam's Garlic Sauce onto his falafel across from me. He said he had something to tell me. All that silent retreating made him realize he was perhaps crazy in love with me? No. He had "met the most wonderful woman" that week in a coffee shop, talked for hours, exchanged numbers, and just had "this feeling" about her that he hadn't felt in a "really long time."

The munchkins froze and then started jamming their pitchforks into my bowels, which I responded to by performing my own nonsurgical, self-induced eye lift. "That's so great, Keith," I lied. "*So great!*" I tried to remember which muscles it took to make my lips curve upward into a smile rather than droop wide open into a gaping look of horror. This wasn't good. This wasn't according to plan.

But hadn't this been my hope for him the entire time I knew him? I needed to lend him my full support. Besides, I rationalized, I was in the throes of my dietetic internship anyway, so time for a relationship would likely be close to impossible. I had renal diets to attend to and large blocks of government-subsidized cheese to dispense to low-income women and their children. "I cannot wait to hear what happens," I told him. I went home and drank way too much green tea kombucha.

After another week, the pressure cooker of emotion, confusion, and the image of coffee-shop girl taking my rightful place in Keith's romantic history continued to bubble and boil in my brain. I decided it was time to release the munchkins wreaking havoc on my insides. We'd had dinner with our mutual friend Seth, during which the two of them reveled in the run-in with coffee-shop girl, now budding into a first date that Friday night with the potential of clothing removal. After their big high-five good-bye and promise of a call or e-mail post–coffee-shop girl date, I asked Keith if he could help me with a broken windshield wiper on my new car. We sat outside Seth's house in my biodiesel VW Golf watching the wiper that had been inexplicably wagging nonstop for three weeks (a mechanical metaphor for my heart, perhaps?) After no more than three minutes of examination, he magically pressed some button or lever and the wagging ceased. As we sat there in the absence of the wiper's hum and click, I inhaled and prayed to the Broccoli Gods.

"Can I ask you something?" I asked, my little heart pulsating with fear. "Do you ever think *we* should be dating?"

Now it was Keith's turn for a nonsurgical eye-lift moment, although since he was a Buddhist, his was far more sedate than mine, and he wasn't wearing mascara. There was a brief but earsplitting silence, after which he calmly stated with an unusual glint in his eye, "Uh, yes, the thought has crossed my mind."

The conversation began, speckled with "What about Todd...what about our friendship...what about coffee-shop girl?" and ending with "Let's just think about it without deciding anything."

I thought about it a *lot*—especially while Keith continued to pursue and date coffee-shop girl. I had been hell-bent on getting him action for the past few years, so it wasn't fair to deny him the opportunity now, even if I preferred that it be with me. Like a true friend and mature adult, I supported his budding relationship. Finally, after weeks of patient waiting, it turned out that coffee-shop girl was just...coffee-shop girl, and Keith and I (green-tea girl) found ourselves awkwardly smooching and holding hands like nervous teens on my purple couch after gulping down a bottle of wine, the sole purpose of which was to blur the lines of friendship. It felt a bit like playing a game of "Spin the Bottle" where the bottle kept landing on the same person, necessitating the "Well, I guess we should just kiss again!"

It took a while, but we slowly transitioned from platonic pal-dom to full blown couple-hood, with many bumps along the way, including my wondering what I should do about all the dirt he now knew about me that I would never have dreamt of sharing with anyone until at least month ten. Maybe he'd forgotten that story I told him about rummaging through the desk drawers of one of my old flames, or the time I had a meltdown that also involved a totally irrational forty-five-minute analysis when a guy I dated just never called me back. Also, sometimes it was just plain weird. We'd be at the same restaurants and movie theatres we had gone to as buddies, except now I was wearing eye shadow and my good bra. And who paid for dinner? We also realized that friends might not always leave parties together, but couples usually do, or should. And that first shower together? It just felt like we wound up there by mistake. *Whoops! Didn't mean to walk in on you. Oh, that's right, we decided to come in here together.*

Turns out OkCupid (and everyone else who spent time with us) was right about the 94 percent chance that we'd be a good match. So good, in fact, that fourteen months in (yes, I am still in seventh grade and count months), we decided to shack up. Kitchens combined (we now had twenty-three random mugs we'd each salvaged from the Goodwill pile), closet space merged ("Wait, are those *your* SmartWool socks or *mine?*"), and decisions about how much we spent weekly on my favorite superfoods, spirulina and maca, were now made as a unit. (*"How* much is an ounce of maca?") He wasn't quite as enamored of the choca-maca lattes I had become accustomed to making regularly, although eventually he came around, thank heavens. And I learned to label all soy in the

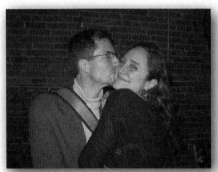

fridge with "Not for Keith," which was successful except for the time when I forgot that soy sauce contains soy. Whoops. We made kale smoothies together, sipped green tea every morning, made meals that frequently included avocados, kale and quinoa, and consistently noticed when the other got a haircut.

The Glory of Green Tea

Oh, tea—or shall I call you *Camellia sinensis*, you lovely leaf, you! Every day around noon, the melancholy drifts over me as I realize the time has come to stop drinking my green tea for the day, since the caffeine (however slight) seems to keep me up at night if I imbibe post-noontime. But for the hours before, I languish in the steeped grassy goodness of this miraculous beverage, which warms, soothes, and strengthens.

In addition to having around sixty milligrams of caffeine per cup, green tea contains the helpful amino acid L-Theanine—also found in chamomile tea—which has been shown to help synthesize calming neurotransmitters in the brain and reduce stress. So, tea drinkers get a mini burst of focused energy as well as a grounding, feel-good shot of calm. There is also a vast amount of research boasting green tea's highly protective compounds called *catechins* that may aid in detoxification, boost immune function, reduce inflammation, and have the potential to reduce the risk of cancer cell growth.* What a perfect package of awesomeness steeped in healthiness! Other studies have shown that green tea can enhance metabolism, boost brain function, and even aid in preventing dental caries. Wowsa—all that from a few little leaves steeped in 175-degree water for a minute or two!**

My favorite green tea happens to be Japanese "Sencha," which I experience as crisp, clean, not too bitter, and with a hint of fresh-cut grass. I know it may not sound entirely appealing to drink grass, unless you are a cow (and if you are, welcome! How did you get access to a computer?), but I can testify that it has a cleansing quality to it that feels like it's mopping your innards.

My tips if you are a newcomer:

---

* Some studies show it can actually turn off cancer promoting genes.

** Ok, most of the research looks at consuming at least a *few* cups of the verdant potion, but still.

- Be careful with drinking green tea on an empty stomach. It can sometimes make the tea novice feel a little woozy. Try it as a midmorning concoction.

- Do not—I repeat, *do not*—oversteep, as the tea will be bitter and you may curse my name and question my credibility.

- If you can buy tea in loose leaf form from a good-quality vendor/ teahouse, that's usually the best way to experience these bits of submerged foliage. Don't feel like leaving your home to wander the streets for a quaint little teahouse with an overly caffeinated or way too Zen tea-o-phile? I've got your back (and your cancer genes). Sugimoto America has an online shop at http://sugimotousa.com/.

- If you get the real stuff, do not fail to get a good tea strainer (not a tea ball or that thingy that looks like two spoons making out with each other). If you must buy a bagged team here are a few brands that I think are pretty decent: A Mighty Leaf, Republic of Tea, and the Jasmine Green Numi Teas. Stay clear of Lipton, Tazo, Stash, or Bigelow brand green teas, which essentially taste like the tea bags they come in.

- Start with a one-minute steep and make sure the water is not boiling, which can damage the tea leaves and reduce their healthy potential. If the grassy thing doesn't do it for you, try a flavored green tea. Some teas come with a peachy or other fruity flavor, which can add a touch of subtle sweetness. Be sure to have a little sniff beforehand; otherwise, you might end up feeling like you are drinking you grandmother's sachet, and nobody enjoys that.

- You can also skip the steep completely and go for *matcha*, a finely ground powder of green tea leaves. This just requires adding hot water (not boiling!) to one teaspoon of matcha and sipping slowly while thanking me in your head. Add a touch of honey and perhaps a splash of your favorite milk-like substance, and you'll be writing a letter thanking me via pen and paper. Try a sprinkle of cinnamon atop that, and you might just nominate me for Outstanding Dietitian of the Year!

(Thank you. I accept.) If you don't like it, it wasn't me. Please note, this tends to be higher in caffeine because you are consuming the leaves in their entirety and not throwing them away in your compost bin. You have a compost bin, right?

Try a cup of green tea today and join those of us who hail it as an elixir of health! If you have discovered a creative way to include green tea in your drinks and/or meals, please don't keep these ideas to yourself! Email me.* The more ways I can learn about how to enjoy green tea, the better I believe my life will be.

References: https://www.ncbi.nlm.nih.gov/pmc/articles/PMC2855614/

---

* See the *Mary's Nutrition Show* episode "Terrific Teas": https://www.youtube.com/marypurdy.

VEGETABLES AND YOU: A LOVE STORY, WAITING TO HAPPEN

A fraid of a little rutabaga? Nervous about beets? Confused by cauli-flower? Or do you find yourself lamenting, "I just don't *like* or have time to make vegetables"? Well, I'll be candid. I'm sick of it. That's right. Prepare for a minor talking to.

#1. It's time to stop thinking that eating vegetables and, God forbid, *cutting* vegetables is some sort of time-consuming hardship. If I had a carrot for every time I heard someone talk about how difficult it is to chop veg-etables, honestly, I would have a cauldron of carrot soup. Grabbing a knife from a knife block and placing a vegetable on a wooden cutting board and then moving one's wrist up and down to cut that tuber into chunks will take less than three minutes, and—extra bonus—it can burn a few calories! I haven't looked into the exact numbers, but I'm going to guess-timate that it should burn at least seventeen calories depending on how enthusiastic you get. (Side note: When I chop kale, I burn at least twenty-two calories, as I am also dancing at the same time in great anticipation.)

Many folks are often barking about how there just isn't enough time for physical activity. Here's an opportunity to get closer to eating an increased amount of vegetables and exercise a bicep at the same time! Plus, I have mentioned before the cathartic pleasure of hacking a potato. What's that? You don't have the time to lift up a knife and slice, dice, or grate? Well, the time that it takes you to complain about the time you don't have is the same amount of time it will take you to cut that vegetable. Quick! Say, "I have no time. I'm too busy." (Your turn. Say it out loud: "I have no time. I'm too busy.") I just made two chopping movements in that time. I'm halfway through a pepper. And I burned 4.6 calories.*

#2. Ok, so I got you to cut the vegetable, but now comes the "Boring. It's just a vegetable. There's no flavor. Where's my bacon cheeseburger with sizzlin' onions?" First of all, a good quality cucumber that has not been waxed and sitting in the vegetable market for seventeen days is deliciously complete with a simple sprinkle of salt and pepper or a dash of paprika.** If you don't think so, it might be time to purchase a tongue scraper to get that crap off your tongue so you can actually taste stuff. And if you've never had an avocado with a splash of lime juice *solamente*, my friend, you have never tasted perfection! Oh, you disagree? Ok, well, chew on this: how about some blessed chili powder on top of that? Yeah! Now we're talking. Is your mouth watering yet? It should be, because salivary glands are highly stimulated by visual images of foods that are likely to activate them. Think about Sour Patch Kids. *Think about them!* See? Now go back and think about lime juice and a dash of chili powder atop a pillowy avocado. Oh my God, I just slobbered on the computer keyboard. I apologize.

#3. What about that energy you're always hoping to have more of? Allow me to introduce you to…vegetables, the consumption of which allows you to ingest more vitamins and minerals, and the lack of which is contributing to that midafternoon energy dip, the occurrence of which sends you wandering over to Shirley's candy jar at work. In case you were sleeping in your seventh-grade science class, plants (a.k.a. vegetables) sit around all day (those lazy bums!) photosynthesizing energy from the sun. Therefore, when we eat them, what do we get? Yuppity yup yup: energy.

Are you fired up yet? No? Need more inspiration for cooking those veggies? Ok, have you ever heard of an onion (like the "sizzlin'" ones that christen that cheeseburger you were yappin' about!) or seen a clove of garlic lingering around your kitchen? These are your friends. They

---

* This is an estimated energy expenditure and has not been scientifically proven. Nor will it ever be. Which is too bad, because I think this could really help people eat more vegetables.

** See the *Mary's Nutrition Show* episode "Will Salt Kill Me?": https://youtu.be/ fUkkP4gXFXE

will set you free from your vegetable inertia. Toss either or both into a pan with olive oil alongside side your freshly chopped veggies, and you just turned into Martha Stewart.

What's that? Onions make your eyes water? Garlic makes your hands smell...like...garlic? You know what I smell? The smell of excuses, my veggie-fearing friend, and it stinks a lot more than that antioxidant-rich bulb. Quit with the jaw-flapping and get a head start on your adventure in the produce world. Grab a knife, or get familiar with the reason you were given teeth. Go out and purchase some chives, for God's sake. Invest in a zester. Turn your oven to 400 degrees and place some sliced or diced veggies (or whatever you did with your seventy-two-calorie-busting chopping job) onto a tray with olive oil, a smattering of chives, or the lucky citrus fruit you chose to zest. Your joyful consumption of these, and subsequent postings on social media, will aid toward decreased complaining around the suffering created by the task of vegetable chopping. This means there will be less of that cauldron of carrot soup that I have to freeze. Thank you.

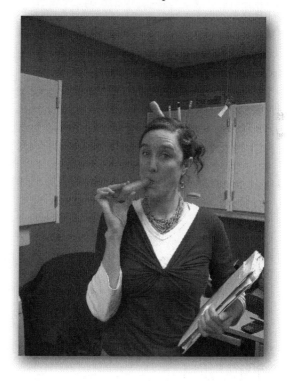

THE BIRTH OF NOURISHING
BALANCE HEADQUARTERS

After completing a yearlong dietetic internship and a rigorous exam where I was able to recall important information like the fact that taking lithium depletes the body of potassium, high-serum albumin indicates possible dehydration, and a #10 spoon in a working kitchen is equivalent to a quarter cup, I was given the sanctioned title of Registered Dietitian. I had always loathed the eight-to-five work schedule (which I had adhered to for nine months in the internship) and wanted full autonomy in my life and vacation schedule. I also needed to be able to take a 10:45 a.m. yoga class and not wait until five in the evening to call my East Coast friends who were putting their kids to bed just as I was getting off work in my Pacific-time life.)

So, with very little business savvy and a name whose Google search turned up a couple reviews of shows that I had done in New York City— including my one-woman show *Purdy Woman*, a musical entitled *The High Heeled Women*, and a "Cultural Celebration" event on Manhattan Plaza that I have no recollection of being a part of, I thought it would be wise to start a private nutrition counseling practice. With those two simple but extremely official letters "RD" to the right of my surname, I felt sure the sick and kale-curious masses would soon show. With both confidence and determination, I decided to hang my shingle in the first space that would have me: a four-by-four utility closet at a local gym that I turned into a tiny little office festooned with foodie photos clipped from old 2006/2007 wall calendars, a rickety file cabinet of nutrition education handouts, and a large wooden shelf stacked with messily labeled beans and grains in jars. Happily, the year before grad school, I had enrolled in an online certificate-mill "Holistic Health Counseling" program that outfitted me with a ready-made website, so I input the new address of my gym cubbyhole, submitted my application to the Washington Department of Health, bought a business license, and became Seattle's "Nourishing Balance."

I shared the common space just outside ~~the utility closet~~ my private practice headquarters with two bulky personal trainers, who were constantly eating large pails of steamed chicken and complaining about my presence in their space.

"What are you bringing in now?" one asked, rolling her eyes, as I lugged in a batik tapestry and a small water feature (a jade-colored ceramic bowl with trickling water) that a woman in my networking group who specialized in fêng shui suggested I add to the room.

"Just a little something to block out the grunting noises from the weight room," I responded, smiling.

I hired two interns—graduate students attending the same program I had completed the year prior—and put them to work with creating corporate wellness brochures, designing flyers for the free "Sugar, Skin, and You" workshop I was going to give in the Pilates studio at the gym (seven people attended, thank you very much, two of whom were Keith's sister-in-law and her friend). I gave dozens of free lectures and presentations at community centers, hospitals, and long-term care facilities, slowly building my mailing list and clientele along the way.

I'd meet people at events and parties who'd ask me, "So what do you do?" When I replied, "I'm a dietitian/nutritionist," they'd respond with, "Oh, well, I had oatmeal for breakfast this morning."

"Ok," I'd say. "Thank you for letting me know." And they'd ask me for my card.

"I'm totally going to call you. I could use your help." Do you think they ever did? You are right. Nope. Oatmeal clearly solves all problems.

I signed on to take insurance, which broadened the patient population who could utilize my services for free or a small copay, which was fantastic for them but, depending on the insurance company, sometimes meant a check for a paltry thirty-seven dollars arrived in the mail for the dedicated hour I spent with someone helping to start the reversal of their prediabetes. (Thanks, Premera Blue Cross Health Insurance!) But no matter. I had passion! I had drive! I had grit! I had lived in New York City! If I could make it there, I'd make it. Wait—I *hadn't* made it there! Hmm. Well, if I *almost* made it there, I could make it in Seattle!

With a dozen more live presentations and my "*almost* made it in New York" status, I started getting a reputation for speaking and was lining up paid gigs and gaining a larger clientele. I gradually moved office locations (I know, shocking that I wouldn't want to stay in the broom closet with those chicken-breath hulks), first to a huge, sun-filled, yet super-cozy space filled with wonderfully pudgy red leather couches and lush potted plants that I shared with two massage therapists and an energy healer; then joining forces with one of my old professors at a clinic filled with physicians and health practitioners where I made my happy health-promoting home for six years, and then finally to the clinic associated with my graduate school, Bastyr Center for Natural Health, which felt like landing a part in the Broadway show I had always hoped to be cast in. It was bright, bike-able, and filled with like-minded naturopathic practitioners, some of whom I had idolized as a student. Even the receptionists were drinking kombucha.* I had come full circle. I knew the Broccoli Gods were cheerfully watching as I gathered my patients from the waiting room, sat them down in my office, and asked, "How can I help you today?"

---

* See the *Mary's Nutrition Show* episode "Gut Health: Fermentation, Probiotics, and How to Make Your Gut Happier": https://youtu.be/wJQSk4ArOzA

WHEN RECIPES CHANGE YOUR DNA

I need to tell you something. Come closer and keep it quiet, will you? This is for you and your ears and eyes only. Pay no attention to the other folks possibly reading this book. It's you and me on this page right now. Get it? Ok, don't tell anyone, but despite the fact that I have been a diehard foodie and subsequent clinical nutritionist, I never had the slightest interest in cooking. I was the queen of throwing things together to make a balanced and healthy meal (that usually included kale and some kind of grain that gets stuck in your teeth) but nothing close to a dish you might serve to friends without apologizing. There were only a handful of times that I cooked for others or held a dinner party throughout all of my twenties (I believe I made a chicken roast once that was edible) and the majority of my thirties (I mostly ate out or grabbed vittles from the natural market's salad and hot bars.)

I just couldn't be bothered. Cooking seemed like a total waste of the time. Like every other person who has ever lived in this century, I was "too busy." Besides, I was a perpetual rookie in the kitchen: burning brown rice, undercooking winter squash, and destroying stews and soups with a surplus of salt and a famine of flavor. To avoid the shame and shock, I hid my lackluster skills well by not inviting people over for dinner.

In New York City (pre-nutritionist but still a health nut), my excuse was easy and a common complaint: "My kitchen is basically a closet with no counter space," I'd say. (This was 100 percent true, but I can think of about twenty-seven cookbook authors who maintained success under such circumstances.) Living in Manhattan also meant that there was an Indian bistro on the corner, a Thai joint down the street, a Chinese restaurant up the street, and about four twenty-four-hour delis within a two-block radius. Who needed to cook? I ate out, ordered in, and relied on my staples: smoothies, mushroom and spinach omelets with feta, veggie couscous with feta, and pasta with tomato sauce and...feta. Feta had an undeniable way of making anything it touches taste like the "Mediterranean Special" on a restaurant menu. I never had to apologize about feta—unless, of course, I had forgotten to add it.

I had over a dozen unopened recipe books taking up precious space in my kitchen, given to me by well-intentioned family members and friends ("Mary loves vegetables, so surely she'll cook nonstop out of this *101 Ways to Cook Cauliflower!*") All of them had pristine pages, lacking the smudges and smidges of tomato paste, olive oil, and maple syrup that grace the pages of the books of real chefs who actually use them. Occasionally, I'd cut out a recipe from a magazine, the plan being to dazzle friends with culinary creations I felt I would and *should* make, but they usually wound up in a crumpled ball at the bottom of my bag, stuck to the remnants of a spirulina sesame ball I purchased at the local twenty-four-hour deli.

One would imagine that moving to the foodie heaven of Seattle and attending a nutrition grad school that had its own "Whole Foods kitchen"—with counter space for fifteen cooks, every kitchen gadget you could dream of, and a curriculum designed to inspire you to cook— would have immediately turned me into a fervent chef whizzing around the kitchen in my "Eat More Kale" apron, concocting the very items I had learned about in my "Bioactive Compounds" class that day.* But no. Meal prep was a chore and not something I looked forward to after a full day of thinking hard, learning, memorizing glycolysis, and applying

---

* Bioactive compounds are extranutritional constituents (as in, not necessary for survival but still really important) that typically occur in small quantities in foods and which may or may not impart health and antioxidant benefits. Doesn't that sound awesome? We're talking about things like anthocyanins found in eggplant that may prevent Alzheimer's! Don't you want to go out and make a ratatouille? Yeah, I didn't either. See my mini "Ode to Phytochemicals," which are examples of bioactive compounds.

nutrition concepts to mock patients (whom I was encouraging to cook more). The last thing I wanted to do was think *more*, when I could just smile at the deli dude at the Natural Foods Coop and say, "I'll have the Emerald City Fennel Salad and the Turkish Apricot Chickpea Dish, please!" Voila! Dinner was served.

But then...something changed. Was it getting married? (Yup, I married Keith.) Buying a house with a real kitchen that had a nook? (Yes, a nook! A perfect little spot to share secrets and play footsie with your partner over a home-cooked meal!) Shifting how I perceived the use of time or meal preparation prioritization? (Maybe I'm *not* too busy to cook!) Perhaps a mixture of all of the above? Whatever the case, at the age of forty-four, I began to feel an unfamiliar sense of longing to cook and create. I grew oddly enthusiastic about recipes. (People are just so darn creative! Vegan Avocado Chocolate Mousse with Olive Oil? Come *on!*) and started baking, braising, and broiling as a way to *relax.* (Chopping helped as well. Nothing like hacking at a large tuber to get out your aggressions.)

The cooking gene that I thought had been missing in my genomic sequencing began to express itself. Similar to women who suddenly feel their biological clocks ticking (something that has never happened to me), I had a "chef-ternal" instinct kick in that made my cooking timer go off. I think my taste buds started lactating.

I brought out of hiding a stack of old unread *Vegetarian Times* magazines and started flipping through the pages. Their recipes chanted to me until I gingerly ripped them from their bindings, began rummaging around for the ingredients in my pantry, and didn't stop until I pulled my Tofu Enchiladas and Baked Yam Chips from the oven. (See? You *should* save all those magazines in your basement. It is entirely possible that you will look at them one day, despite what your judgmental partner with a totally uncluttered desk thinks.)

I would wind down at night by organizing the recipes into an alphabetically organized binder, putting broccoli dishes under *B* and salmon under *S*. (This occasionally got complicated when there was a salmon-broccoli dish and I had to Xerox the recipe and scribble on the top, "*See*

71

also Salmon.") The binder grew fat with possibility as I imagined myself dancing around the kitchen with each ingredient, my toes grasping the spatula to stir the lentil stew (filed under *L*) while my hands chopped the celeriac (filed under *C*). Keith would see the cutouts strewn on the counter by my bedside atop the Nook table.

"When are you making these Chive Chickpea Pancakes?" he'd ask, droplets of saliva pooling in the corners of his mouth.

"I'm not sure," I'd reply. "Tomorrow? This weekend?"

I'll be frank. Sometimes these pages with raging "yum" potential got made, and sometimes they just took up space. (I apologize to Keith for getting his hopes up for pancakes way too many times.)

Then came the deal sealer: *The Cookbook*. This was no ordinary publication. The well-designed cover parading every blessed vegetable imaginable was what initially drew me in. But upon opening this foodie tome, I realized that the content was much more than ingredients to be bought and directions to be followed. Oh no—these recipes were short stories that took me on a mental and physical journey.

I read eagerly about the specifics in "Fennel with a Toasted Sesame Flourish." Honestly, I wasn't sure whether the pairing of these two plants would be successful. Wouldn't the pungent personality of fennel dominate? Might pepitas be a more suitable match? Don't sesame seeds go better with ginger? I quickly learned that, like most relationships, there was sacrifice and compromise to be had. Fennel (with the help of its trusted and tear-jerking companion, the yellow onion) toned down its temperament, honoring the smaller but distinct and lively addition of sesame. And sesame? Well, while still staying true to its nature, sesame allowed the space for fennel to shine and realize its potential. It was clear in the final and tasty outcome that sometimes you have to be willing to give up a part of yourself for the sake of the partnership.

There were other tales about unlikely partners in this juicy novel who also had successful marriages: basil and strawberry; tofu and rosemary; watermelon and my dear old friend feta!

"Did you mean to put these in a bowl together?" Keith would ask.

"Stop judging and wait until the effective coupling starts mingling in your mouth!" I'd snap back while licking the garam masala off my fingers.

I learned about the unexpected and bumpy road that sturdy grain teff took in order to transform into a plate of brownies with the help of her allies cocoa powder, maple syrup, and arrowroot. I wasn't sure if she would make it, but it's amazing what a simple hand mixer and a 375-degree environment can help one achieve.

I couldn't wait to find out about what happened to the rice that got mixed up with a bunch of shredded herbs and purple cabbage in the "Confetti Salad" and was on the edge of my seat waiting to see what pumpkin puree, almond butter, and coconut oil would do when things got heated. I didn't think it would turn out well, but in the end, some fantastic muffins emerged out of the oven. Miraculous. It was as if the cookbook had been written with me in mind. "What might Mary enjoy?" the authors had obviously pondered, and before they knew it, recipes with coconut, cucumber, kale, and kabocha squash were born.

Despite my desire to be some kind of artsy cook who just "wings it" and hopes all goes well, it turned out that following directions almost always leads to a level of success! (Unless you have a shitty recipe. Thanks a lot, *Bon Appetit*, for the forty-five minutes I wasted to make that crappy slop of a mess you titled "Coconut Chile Palapa Sauce." I swear I followed that thing to a T!) There is a reason someone spends hours figuring out the exact amount of cinnamon needed to maintain the tang of a cherry tart.

Keith would sit mouth agape in the dining nook as Coconut Mung Bean Curry made its way onto the table, blazing with steam and unfamiliar, but soon to be adored, flavors. I still did some initial apologizing and tried not to feel hurt when he sprinkled on a tablespoon of extra salt. I admit that I was shy about my skills. Just because you have the passion doesn't mean you have the chops. Even following directions did not seem to place me in the "what a great cook!" category, as much as I tried. I was (and still am) adequate, at best.

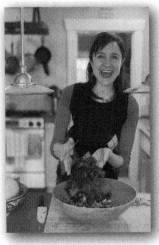 But if singing makes you happy, should you stop doing it even if you cannot keep a tune? So what if the dish wasn't something I'd pay $13.95 for at a restaurant? I couldn't help feeling a sense of accomplishment that I had *made* something whole out of a series of parts. Where there had just been a jar of olives, a few dried figs, and a garlic clove, there was now a mouthwatering tapenade. Setting aside that thirty to forty minutes of time was a simple gift that I gave to myself, where my brain cells were not saturated with e-mails or someone's requests on the other end of the phone. It was just me, the ingredients, and NPR floating on the peaceful raft of a Sunday night.

Friends and family who had heard about my outpouring of succulence sent an abundance of cookbooks my way—including *Ayurvedic Vegan Desserts, 1001 Superfood Soups for the Soul,* and *50 Shades of Kale*—all of which I adored, but I knew that even if I lived to be 100 (which I hoped that eating from these cookbooks would help me to achieve), I would never be able to get through them all, even with my very determined and organized earmarking. (Not to mention the now two enormous notebooks of close to five hundred torn out recipes, of which *maybe* twenty-seven have been created.)*

However, the stage had been set, my brain was rewired, and my fingers—which had rarely gripped a whisk with any enthusiasm—periodically tingled to tackle a polenta cake or a plum-rhubarb crisp. I even bought a Cuisinart and a strange fish-poaching contraption made of questionable materials. I felt I had some baseline skills to match my title even if I had no plans to photograph my flourless chocolate ganache or

---

* Since the initial writing of this essay, I can guarantee you that at least 43 additional recipes have been torn from their magazine hinges and placed into one of the four notebooks on our kitchen shelves.

enter a bean-dip contest. And I had new friends like cardamom, mustard seed, almond flour, and smoked paprika. I still do keep it pretty simple, and I am as much delighted with a slice of salmon and avocado on whole-grain toast that takes less than four minutes to prepare as I am with the Butternut Squash Risotto that takes forty.*

I'm not trying to win any recipe competitions, nor am I expecting to ever hear "Mary, will you please make your famous sweet potato dish for us?"** but I look forward to the day when I stop hearing Keith ask me to "Pass the salt please, babe," with the most loving and earnest expression on his face. Until then, I embrace my status as a "sufficient enough" player in the kitchen, and I will keep reading my one-page novellas, eager to find out how they end.

---

* Full disclosure: There are days when the cooking verve is non-existent and I eat beans straight out of the can, dip salsa into my mouth, munch on two raw carrots, pop a couple nuts and call it good. *Very* good.

** I don't have a famous sweet potato dish. This is just an example, but if you would like to commission me for one, I'm happy to give it my best shot.

Purdy's Ode to Phytochemicals*

Intro to the Ode: Many food groups like fruits and vegetables (and herbs and spices) showcase a color that reflects a high antioxidant content (excepting deceptive items like the red Starburst, which holds no nutritional value, unless children screaming with glee = value, which many decades ago, it did for me.) These antioxidants benefit our bods by essentially reducing inflammation and disarming harmful molecules that arise from exposure to environmental toxins, cigarette smoke, pollution, and the by-products of our own natural metabolism, among other things. Yes! Eek! We actually produce toxins just by being human. Anyhoo, instead of just giving you a list of high-antioxidant foodstuffs and their associated colors, I thought I'd scribble down my personal ode which highlights a few plants in order to showcase these antioxidants with the artistry they deserve. Please note: there are many white plants like onions and cauliflower that should not go unnoticed for their potential cancer ass-kicking prowess, but when you are sticking with the theme of ROYGBIV, the whities get left out. Sorry. Here goes. All phytochemicals have been bolded to indicate their unflinching devotion to keeping you healthy.

Red wraps around the tomato in my salad, speckles my Fuji apple after lunch, blesses the strawberry in my morning smoothie, and gives life to the cranberries in the freezer. It is bold and strong, bursting with **lycopene** waiting to neutralize reactive molecules swarming my body after I sit in traffic for an hour. It reminds me of blood, of flesh that is ripe and vulnerable.

Orange wanders over my peach, shades my apricot, covers my carrot, and bathes my sweet potato in rich tones. The orange is so orange it has stolen the color's name for itself! It is perpetually beta-testing its **beta-carotene** on my immunity. The pumpkin

---

* See the *Mary's Nutrition Show* episode "Why You Need to Eat More Antioxidants": https://youtu.be/R8zn0LumWm8.

makes an advertisement for her pigment every October as she shines in the window presenting her fiery tint.

Yellow ensconces my banana, marries my spaghetti squash, bequeaths itself to the yellow pepper, and takes ownership of the yolk, aspiring to be as bright as it can be, sometimes melding with its auburn sister. It broadcasts its **carotenoids** shimmering like a sunbeam on my blood vessels.

Green emanates from the kale in the garden, oozes out of broccoli stalks and peapods at the farmers market, and drips from the avocado just barely hanging on the branch. It shouts its shades from lime and olive to kelly and emerald, heralding its cancer-fighting **chlorophyll.** Even the simple sprig of cilantro gets a hit.

Blue coats the berries that bear its moniker, canoodles the plum—both fresh and dried—envelops the elderberry, sharing violet's anti-inflammatory **anthocyanin** status but wondering why there aren't more natural hues of itself in the grocery aisles not defined as "dye # 1" on a child's popsicle stick.

Violet is a true friend to the eggplant, passionately defends the blackberry, protects and shrouds the beet, and emblazons itself upon the grape, raging with **resveratrol.** It is known to dot the shirts of those consuming the fruitlets it paints as overzealous bites are taken or napkins go unused.

Reference: https://www.ncbi.nlm.nih.gov/pmc/articles/PMC2841576/.

UNDONE BY A CHEERIO

I was trapped in my small office alone with a blond two-year-old staring at me from a polka-dot stroller. He was the son of my patient who couldn't find childcare this morning for our nutrition counseling appointment.

"Will you watch him for a couple minutes while I run to the bathroom?" she asked, wiping sweet-potato goop off her sweater.

"Sure!" I said. "No problem."

But it was a problem, because I had no idea what to do with a two-year-old for two minutes. I didn't have kids, never wanted them, and mostly equated spending time with toddlers to being on an awkward first date. Meaning, I was eager to see it end. Usually, during these uncoordinated moments, someone else had been around to fill in the blanks, make the faces, and know the latest Legos. Staring back at this tot in Baby Gap's finest, I felt transported into a play whose script I didn't have. My head was a cavern of "I've got nothing."

I spent my days listening to medical histories, exploring eating behaviors, educating on mineral deficiencies, and recommending ways to lower cholesterol and avoid gluten. I had a sea of knowledge of the latest studies on fish oil, turmeric, and avocados, but I was inarticulate at toddler-speak.

Sweat tickled my lower back. I couldn't have my patient return with the two of us gawking at each other. We had to be engaged in some sort of discourse or game. He needed to be giggling or cooing at my entertaining magic show. If she couldn't trust me with a two-year-old, why would she rely on me for medical advice?

"So…how are you?" I asked. He popped another Cheerio in his mouth. "How are you?" always released a floodgate from my usual clientele, but I doubted its effectiveness as an opening gambit for this demographic.

"I like your plaid shirt!" I offered.

He looked down at his plaid shirt but expressed little interest in the shirt or me. I looked around my office for child-friendly conversation starters. The framed painting of a radish, two office chairs, copious nutrition textbooks, and jars of grains and beans didn't offer a shred of help in transforming me into Dr. Seuss.

I grabbed a food model off my shelf and gently shook it up and down.

"Look, it's a box of gluten-free pasta!" I said, holding it like a puppet bouncing back and forth.

"Look at me!" I continued, imitating what I thought sounded like Kermit the Frog's voice. "I'm gluten-free pasta! Dum dee dum dum dum." He stared. There was a desert of sound.

"Isn't this a nice logo?" I said, my normal voice shaking with effort. "And it's super yummy! Do you like pasta?"

He nodded cautiously. Progress. Quick, keep going, I urged myself.

"Pasta, pasta!" I sang, channeling Ella Fitzgerald.

I started googling my brain to remember what they sang about on *Sesame Street* in the '70s. Did they ever talk about vegetables? Should I start reciting the alphabet? Crooning about numbers? Might he be interested in reading over some blood labs with me? "Look at this high cholesterol. Can you say '243'?" My patient must have been finished in the bathroom by now! She said "a couple minutes," but I had been stuck here babbling about noodles for a half hour. While I scrambled to find a captivating box of high-fiber crackers, my patient reentered the room, shirt free of all tuber remnants.

"Thanks for watching him," she said

"Sure!" I squeaked, and the two-year-old shifted in his stroller. He had my number. He knew I'd panicked. Thank God he still had limited vocabulary and couldn't reveal my fumblings. I made a mental note to myself to watch *Bob the Builder*, go to the Legos website, and Google "how to speak with two-year-olds" in preparation for next time. I began the session with my patient and relaxed into adult conversation.

"So, tell me how things are going for you," I began. As she launched into her list of challenges around IBS and anemia, I thought, "Ah yes, *this*, I can handle." I saw her son eyeing me, surely wondering what our next encounter would be like. Chances are I'd be dancing around my computer, shaking a bottle of vitamin D pills for percussion and building a sand castle of quinoa as he stared blankly, catching me in my clumsy charade.

WHY I LOVE THE HECK OUT OF GROCERY SHOPPING

I adore grocery shopping. One of my ideal ways to spend a Saturday night is lingering amid the lemons, ambling around the apples, perusing the pickles, and zoning out by the zucchini. Shopping for food is more like a hobby than a chore. It's like a little trip to a food museum, and on a Saturday night, I don't have to rush. I don't have to get back to anything except for…the rest of Saturday night.

Normally, on a quick weeknight shop, I have to stay on the route, focused and predictable, purchasing the necessities: kale, lemons, garlic, cilantro, quinoa, carrots, sweet potatoes, apples, oranges, almonds and sunflower seeds, cans of chick peas and black beans, tortillas, and "Don't forget the salsa," yells Keith. (Or the coconut milk!) I have the list down pat in my head. I know what we need for a typical week of meals so that we've got enough balance, bounty, color, fiber, sweet, sour, plain, and fancy.

But on Saturday night at the Pacific Central Food Coop in Seattle, the world is mine. Sometimes Keith comes along with me on Saturday, and we make a night out of it together. "Shall we do that thing where we have dinner at the grocery store and then do the shopping?" he will ask. It's so romantic.

I luxuriate in the time I can spend reading labels and comparing ingredients, (wow, this brand has guar gum, while this one uses carrageenan!), discovering new products (there are nineteen different brands of mustard!), sneaking a taste of something in the bulk bin (what exactly is in those gritty little chunks of brown-marbled nuttiness?), and looking at products in the freezer that I've never seen (frozen chicken gizzards? Eek!).

It's an adventure *and* I get to take something home afterward! That doesn't happen at a museum. You cannot actually remove anything from a museum without causing a pretty big ruckus. (Trust me: my mom touched a painting once in a museum in New York City and almost got escorted out by a guard.) But grocery stores let you both touch and take items, historical and modern, out of the building and into the comfort of your own pantry, where you can put them on display for your family members and guests, who can look at them and then devour them.

I am also at home in a grocery store. I appreciate the comforting familiarity of what I see as I stroll, like my favorite box of flaxseed crackers peeking at me from the shelf. "I remember those," my tummy chimes. And now, look, they come in new flavors. "Rosemary!" Heavenly! "Savory?" Well, I'll be damned. "Cinnamon Raisin!" Unheard-of! Crackers with cinnamon and raisin in them. Who thinks of these creative combinations?

I clip coupons as a warm up: my grocery shopping foreplay. I don't care if its thirty-five cents, goshdarnit, I'm determined to spend less than I did at the last trip. I get high off of savings. When I start flipping through those little coupon books and realize I have already saved three dollars and haven't even started putting things in my basket, my heart rate starts rising (not in the "your Aunt Thelma has high blood pressure" kind of way, but rather in the "I just won the raffle prize" kind of way.) It's like I am suddenly holding a three-dollar bill in my hand, which makes me feel powerful—not because three-dollar bills don't exist, but because that was three dollars that I got paid for no other reason than I picked up a little booklet of coupons and looked through it. As I hand over the flimsy two-by-four-inch paper cutout to the cashier, I have this gratifying sensation that I just got something for nothing. Basically, someone just gave me sixty-five cents to help me buy a jalapeño hummus that I was going to buy anyway.

I scour the aisles for sales (more savings!)—denoted by a bright orange sign—and grab those items off the shelves with extra spirit. And I'm not too proud to say that yes, I wait for the sales and then buy several tubs/bags/cartons of that item. Bam! Just saved (or made) four dollars and ninety-eight cents. And it's not going to take me all that long to go through those four cartons of almond milk.

On Saturday evenings at my local store, the patrons seem to fall into three categories: First are the market-lovin' foodie folks, coupons peeking out of their pockets (hello, *moi*), taking the time to choose the perfect tomato, studying labels, and relishing a chocolate-covered coconut chunk they snuck from the bulk bin. Yes, that would be *me* again. I admit, I have ~~stolen~~ borrowed and not returned a number of items from this area. I consider it market research—often a chance to test out items that I will likely be buying or recommending to patients, or just to make sure 100 percent for the seventeenth time that I do still, in fact, like tamari-roasted almonds. You just never know if your tastes have changed!

The second category: couples on a dinner-making date, buying the ingredients for their meal—the older ones quibbling, the newer ones trying to be as agreeable as possible. "Um, sure! I'm fine with any of the different types of pasta. *You* choose!" (We all know that's not true. I have been that person and found myself very disappointed with penne when what I really wanted were spirals—the naturally superior choice.) I have also been the couple getting all lovey-dovey in the canned foods section:

"You look so cute next to those artichoke hearts!"

"This label really brings out your eyes."

(Keith and I don't make out *or* quarrel much as we shop, mostly because we divide up the duties and meet at the checkout line, but many a time we end up with the same Emerald City Kraut, Beet Chips, and Theo's Chocolate in both of our carts, and I know I have found my soul mate.)

And the third category: the solo shopper, shoulders slightly hunched, staring blankly at the ice cream in the freezer section. I have also been in category number three, on nights when Mint Galactica Coconut Bliss ice cream appeared to have great potential to solve the world's problems—or at least put them on pause for a moment. Donald Trump (or our current political turmoil of the day) immediately seems insignificant when you're ladling a scoop of Salted Caramel Chocolate Chunk directly onto your tongue. Yeah, even dietitians have moments of stress-eating. We are still human, after all. Those comfort foods do have a mollifying effect both emotionally and physiologically. (Sugar can stimulate the reward center of the brain, which makes you feel, well…rewarded!)

I don't want to give the impression that I don't still have the occasional crazy Saturday night out smoking hookahs and going to a hard-rock concert. I do. (Minus the hookah, and ok, exchange "hard rock" for "singer-songwriter" at an intimate tavern on a quiet street in a quaint part of town.) There are times, I admit, when I wonder if the comfort in this familiar weekly task has become complacency. Is it true fulfillment in a hearty shop that I feel or just relief and contentment with something easy and familiar? I believe I've learned to find delight (or perhaps accept the delight that I naturally feel) in a simple evening of mingling with the miso paste at the community market, but I'm sometimes left wondering if I spent more time poring through the coupon booklet than I did perusing the "Things to Do in Seattle This Week" section of the paper. I tell myself that when you feel connected to food, spending precious time with it feels less like a chore and more like a gift that offers culture, entertainment, and experiential learning—especially when you partake of as much "secret sampling" as I do. And I usually can find parking. Yet, when I realize that my answer to "What did you do this weekend?" is consistently about the various food-themed encounters I had, I am left scratching my head with the self-query: "Have I become dull?" Or did my kindergarten teacher who wrote "Food is very important to Mary" in my report card have my number and predict my entire life from age five? Was there a concert I should have gone to? A parade that would have been *the best time ever*? Have I forgotten that I love karaoke? But Saturday night will come again, and chances are, I'll be at the co-op again, examining the olive bar and dreaming up ways to use the preserved lemons that are on sale.

Avocado and Walnut Duke It Out*

I was at my kitchen sink doing dishes when I overheard Avocado and Walnut at it again.

"Everyone's talking about me," said Avocado. "Haven't you seen the ads? The signs? I'm heart-healthy."

"Well, so am I," bragged Walnut. "I have a 'board' that works for me. That's right, the Walnut Board of California. They've even got materials that they mail out to people."

"Big deal," snapped Avocado. "Ever hear of the Haas Avocado Board? They are all about *me*. I'm also being represented by the California Avocado Commission."

"Well," said Walnut, "I've been mentioned in numerous science journals claiming that not only am I the richest nut source of omega-3 fatty acids that support healthy blood pressure, but eating me regularly helps with weight loss because of my good fats."

"That's great, fatty!" Avocado snorted. "You can pretty much say the same thing about me, you know. I believe I have a few more monounsaturated fats than you do. Plus, you can easily add me to a sandwich or use me in place of mayonnaise."

"So what?" said Walnut. "Can you get sprinkled on top of oatmeal in the morning or baked into a cookie?"

"As a matter of fact," said Avocado, "some folks just started replacing butter in cookies with me. Um, have you ever heard of vegans? So, yes, I make it into cookies periodically, too. I don't believe I've ever seen *you* in a taco."

"Depends on who's making the taco, buddy," snipped Walnut. "Have *you* ever heard of raw foodists? Sometimes they replace the meaty meat in tacos with yours truly, and I get to enjoy the ride in a soft tortilla surrounded by my new pal Pico de Gallo."

"Oh, de Gallo and I hang out like every day," bragged Avocado. "We practically live together! And you know who talks

---

* See the *Mary's Nutrition Show* episode "Fat: Friend or Foe?": https://youtu.be/2-yp0mgjgso

about me a lot? Julia Roberts. Someone pinned one of her break-
fasts, and it included *moi.*"

"Big deal!" shouted Walnut. "I have a theatre company named
after me. The Walnut Street Theatre."

"That's because there's a street named 'Walnut Street' where
the theatre is located!" screeched Avocado.

"Well, I don't see any Avocado Streets or Avenues," harrumphed Walnut.

"For your information, there's one in California. Get around
much?" said Avocado.

"I get around a *lot,*" smirked Walnut. "I've got a street in Philly,
and an avenue in Seattle! Plus, I don't want to lord this over you too
much, but there are more than just streets and avenues named in
my honor. There are places: Walnut Creek, Walnut Grove, Walnut
City."

Avocado paused, fuming. "Well, I hear you're associated with
a lot of allergies."

"So what?" said Walnut. "I'm a tree nut. It's gonna happen."

"Well," said Avocado, "I'd say a pretty small percentage of
the population is allergic or 'sensitive' to me."

"I bet they will be once they start genetically modifying you!"
Walnut jeered.

"They wouldn't dare!" cried Avocado.

I'd had just about enough of this bickering.

"Stop it, you two!" I yelled. "You're both fantastic and have
helped me to improve the health of many a patient!"

"But..." they protested.

"Enough!" I roared. "Yes, Walnut is a great source of omega-3s
and magnesium, and the last article I read showed it helped to
bring down the blood pressure of forty-six overweight adults in
Connecticut."

Walnut glowered.

"Don't get ahead of yourself, Walnut," I said. "Avocado is
a powerhouse of fiber and potassium and was recently featured

in a PowerPoint I watched showing its ability to reduce LDL cholesterol."

Avocado harrumphed.

"It's time you two started getting along. None of this 'I'm better than you are' and 'There's a Podunk town named after me' stuff."

I pulled out a cookbook, turned to page 242, and recited the recipe title aloud: "Avocado Cheesecake with a Walnut Crust."

Avocado and Walnut both gasped.

"When you two work together, it's possible to make something magical," I said.

I grabbed the cutting board and a bowl, and the union began.

Lime and Coconut Oil, who had been listening in from the pantry, said, "Uh, we'd like to help. Is there a place for us in this recipe?"

I smiled. "Of course, there is. You two are going to help bring it all together."

A recipe for you so you can bring it all together too! https://paleoleap.com/chocolate-avocado-mousse-walnut-crust/

References

https://www.ncbi.nlm.nih.gov/pubmed/23756586
http://jaha.ahajournals.org/content/4/1/e001355)

CLINICIAN'S CHART NOTE ON MARY PURDY

Name of Patient: Mary S. Purdy
Sex: Female
DOB 01/25/1970
Height: 5'8"
Weight: 130.6lbs
BMI: 21

R eason for Visit: Subjective Data: Patient's chief complaint is stated as a deficiency of adventure in life, perpetual sensations of FOMO (Fear of Missing Out), chronic drive to succeed, and overall malaise with current predictable weekend activities mostly related to nutrition and food.

Patient reports being happy with professional life as a registered dietitian nutritionist in Seattle, Washington, and having excellent relationship and happy home life with husband of five years, yet feels a longing for what she terms "kooky crazy shit" to occur in order to make her feel as if she is "truly living" and to have more stories to write about and tell friends and fellow bloggers. Periodically feels jealous when hears about friends and family members renting "villas" in Spain or riding elephants in Thailand. Experiences a sense of angst when people quote the Mary Oliver poem, "Tell me, what is it you plan to do with your one wild and precious life?"

Expresses guilt over this sense of dissatisfaction since patient knows that she is blessed with being a "privileged white American" and should probably "just be grateful that I have it this good and am not in a war-torn territory, or living in rural America married to a polygamist with seventeen kids."

Six years ago, Patient took trapeze classes, which made her feel like she was getting "out of her comfort zone," but had to stop due to torn rotator cuff. Has done a fair amount of travelling but no recent "wild escapades" in the jungle, mountains, or back streets of Bavaria as she has hoped or expected with "white privileged American" status. Often feels compelled to stay in Seattle proper and attend "nutrition-y events" like farmers markets, cultural foodie festivals, and the occasional nutrition conference so she can excel at current profession.

Describes a need to branch out into activities that will make her feel comfortably uncomfortable. Afraid she will reach ninety years old and not have taken more risks. Patient not interested in experiences that she believes may be life-threatening like bungee jumping, beekeeping, or having a child. Cannot seem to identify specifics around what she is looking for but knows that the safe way she is living right now "ain't it." Asks, "How many more farm-to-table events and tea carnivals am I supposed to go to?"

Energy Levels: High with periodic dips. "Even when I'm low energy, I'm high energy. I eat a lot of kale and spirulina." Takes a B complex daily; dubious about the research fully supporting the claims yet feels compelled to continue purchasing the supplement.** Sometimes "does cayenne pepper shots" which help. Currently writing a book of essays for which she has no time and which she feels has a tendency to deplete her energy levels and make her "wonder what it's all for." Doesn't believe anyone will actually read book and already mourning time lost writing it when she should have been volunteering at a Woman's Refugee Center instead.

Stress Levels: Fairly low with a tendency toward high circumstantially. Patient reports that she works on weekends and tends to necessary minutiae like laundry folding, counter wiping, and CD reorganization

---

* See the *Mary's Nutrition Show* episode "10 Powerful Dietary and Herbal Supplements": https://youtu.be/coGXlloZNyI.

instead of taking day- and weekend-long trips to small towns with rivers in which she could swim, mountains she could hike, and goats that she could try to pet. Suffers from ongoing belief that there is "never enough time" despite feeling good at time management and being an avid fan of books *The Four Hour Work Week* and *Getting Things Done.*

Sleep: Ok, with exception of days when patient consumes too much Japanese green tea post 1:00 p.m. or wakes at 3:00 a.m. thinking about villas in Spain and elephants in Thailand. "I really enjoy being awake." Often worries about not getting enough sleep and regularly in bed with ear plugs in and eye mask on by 10:00 p.m., which may contribute to her avoiding risky or adventurous escapades. However, claims that poor sleep will result in even further distancing from said escapades, as energy will not be available to fuel these capers. Patient cocked head and asked, "Chicken or the egg?"

Diet: "Excellent." Patient makes diet a priority and happily eats high volume of healthy whole foods that often get stuck in her teeth. Specifies that "whole foods" does not refer to the grocery store chain Whole Foods but rather to foods like fruits, vegetables, nuts, seeds, beans, and whole grains that have not been significantly altered by machines or injected with random genes from the zebra fish. Is willing to try almost anything provided it isn't highly processed or detrimental to one's health or the environment. "I have eaten crickets, rabbit, goat, and elk," but doesn't plan to do so again. Hates mayonnaise and zucchini. Currently "obsessed" with mulberry tea and avocados. Becomes a "whirling dervish" if consumes coffee.

Doesn't believe in germs and is at ease with eating food that has fallen on the ground or dirty floor. Patient claims that as a two-year-old she licked the floor of the airport in Kabul, Afghanistan, when travelling there with her parents and feels this strengthened her immune system. Has no recollection of this adventure but it is now family lore. Patient remains curious about the fearlessness with which she approached this act as a toddler and wonders where that bravery has gone.

Objective: Patient is a 47-year-old female. 5'8" and 130.6 pounds. (Normally at 128 pounds. Patient attributes the recent weight gain to either "muscle development" resulting from more frequent hip-hop dance classes or perhaps just "47-year-old butt and hip spread.") Blood labs all within normal ranges. Blood pressure is at low end of normal at 96/59, which patient reports as usual for her. "Sometimes I see fuzzy little dots when I get up and need to hold the side of the wall to prevent myself from falling." Side note: According to Patient, having low blood pressure that causes her to feel as if she might fall does not constitute the kind of "kooky crazy shit" she is seeking.

Clinical Observations: Healthy, well nourished, middle-aged woman. (Although patient referred to this as the "first third of her life.") Very engaged, cheerful, and energetic. Continually quoted Eleanor Roosevelt's "The purpose of life is to live it, to taste experience to the utmost." Eyes lit up upon the mention of mushroom harvesting and outdoor movies. Pupils dilated when there was mention of "camping outdoors." Heart rate unremarkable until patient stood up to show interesting choreography from her hip-hop class, mostly in an effort to "help make me more memorable to the medical establishment so I'm not just a number in the system." Reflexes normal, although difficult to differentiate between actual reflex and hip-hop dance move.

Clinical Assessment

1. Patient suffers from perceived inadequate adventure in life and classic case irrational "The I Should Bes," related to professed lack of time and current feelings around her life being "predictable" and "not as exciting as someone who works for the Peace Corps or Cirque de Soleil."

2. Patient overly driven to succeed in chosen profession, resulting in delusional notion that all recreational pastimes and pursuits need to be centered around nutrition concepts and cuisine in order for her to advance professionally, fully understand nutrigenomics and the microbiome, and receive recognition as a "outstanding dietitian of the year."

3. Patient appears healthy and somewhat normal, but overeager to find more stimulating experiences in what appears to be an already fairly satisfying and interesting life. Presents as ardently passionate about food yet convinced that free time is supposed to be spent on more wild adventures that go beyond spending her Saturday night at the local grocery store. Grappling with being at peace with this side of herself while also challenging whether this mundaneness truly makes her happy.

Care Plan: Worked with patient on ways she might seek out healthy adventures in her life without causing cardiac arrhythmia, which patient fears. Explored patient's definition of adventure and a "life worth living" in order to better assess exactly what seems to be missing. Provided patient with map of Seattle parks as well as a course catalogue for North Seattle Community College and pointed out various classes that may be of interest and serve as temporary antidote for her desire for travel: Conversational Italian, Cooking with Seaweed, and Survey of Astronomy. Encouraged patient to continue exploring getting out of comfort zone both physically and mentally without compromising rotator cuff or professional development. (Encouraged adhering to the recommendation of attending no more than two nutrition conferences per year, unless one happens to be taking place at a villa in Spain.) Advised against returning to the Kabul airport to relive her floor-licking experience as a toddler. Also discussed the possibility of "glamping," which caused no apparent pupil dilation.

    Handouts Provided: REI catalogue, two Huffington Post articles on "Taking Risks" and "Accepting Where You Are," and recipe for cricket tacos in case Patient changes mind about eating grasshoppers again.

    Follow-Up Ideas: Further explore the meanings of adventure and success. Discuss meditation. Encourage patient to sign up for Groupon Getaways. Investigate Patient's willingness to try herbal and rooibus tea to decrease caffeine load. Rule out parasites.

Cayenne Pepper Shots Take Cojones

Hello, brave soul. You are here to learn the way of the cayenne pepper shot. This was my lifesaver in graduate school when I started drooping at 6pm and knew I still had a full night of studying ahead. There was no way a caffeinated beverage was going to provide anything other than a miserable night of sleep, so I implemented this strategy instead.* I'm not totally sure how I got the idea. Why would someone elect to swallow cayenne pepper without having it immersed in a chili or stew? It may have been the research I was looking at around the possible beneficial effects of capsaicin, the active compound in cayenne, on cancer. I also tend to be quite experimental, if you hadn't noticed. While other members of my class were out having a cocktail, I was in my kitchen concocting my personal witch's brews. (Sans the eye of newt.)

Here it is, plain and simple:

Place 1/8 teaspoon of cayenne pepper in 2 oz of water. Take a deep breath. Grab your cojones or tighten your ovaries and shoot that baby back. *Will it burn?* Um. Yes, a little. But in an invigorating way. (It may also clear your nostrils, my allergy sufferers!) Cayenne acts as a great blood circulant and has the potential to give you that little extra kick in the pants which you might need when you.

Important note: If you are suffering with mouth sores, a raw sore throat, any kind of gastric distress, heart burn or ulcers, I would definitely not advise trying out the cayenne pepper shot. It may aggravate those conditions and compel you to write me a nasty email. However, if your internal mucosal lining is in good condition, give it a go. After the initial shock, you may just feel like jumping on a trampoline or riding an elephant in Thailand.

---

* See the *Mary's Nutrition Show* episode "Sleep Better": https://youtu.be/sW3PSNrhLK4

POST SCRIPT: Here's to wishful thinking...

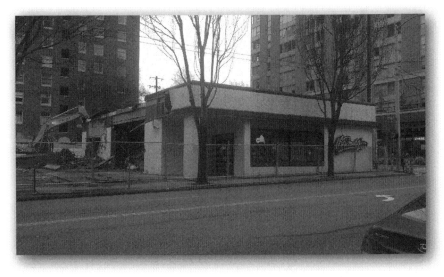

About the Author

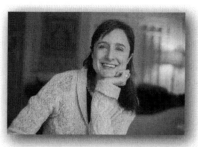

Mary Purdy, MS, RDN, grew up in New York City and spent twelve years as a writer and actor before becoming a registered dietitian. She holds a master's degree from Bastyr University, where she also worked as an adjunct professor and clinical supervisor.

Purdy has been chair of Dietitians in Integrative and Functional Medicine and past president of the Greater Seattle Dietetic Association, and she has given dozens of nutritional presentations to a variety or professional organizations. Today Purdy works as a dietitian and clinical trainer for the scientific wellness company Arivale and lives in Seattle with her husband, with whom she hosts the web series and podcast *Mary's Nutrition Show.*

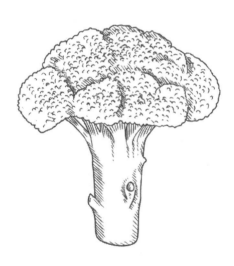

Made in the USA
Columbia, SC
21 May 2020